Mass Delusion

100 Low-carb Lifestyle Secrets

Richard Leach & Justin Whittaker

The Leach Press
'Sportsview'
20 Moor Lane
Nottingham
NG9 3FH
United Kingdom

© The Leach Press

Acknowledgements

First and foremost, we would like to thank all the people that have trusted our off-the-wall assertions and tried low-carb. Without them, we would be lone voices.

Justin would like to nostalgically thank Richard for spamming his Facebook page with high-fat, low-carb facts. At the time Justin thought it the ravings of a madman, and decided to prove him wrong. He failed.

Thanks to Kim Whittaker for cooking and writing up the low carb recipe ideas. Thanks to Danielle Macdonald for helping us with the table of contents, Campbell Mckee for formatting the tables, Patrick Baird for giving us material and advice on fats, and Ed Palmer for doing the final proof.

Of course, none of these ventures are ever possible without the support of family, so love to Sharmin Leach for making the switch with Richard and likewise Kim Whittaker with Justin.

'I cannot teach anybody anything. I can only make them think'

— Socrates

Introduction

A few years ago, Richard Leach uncovered a conspiracy. A conspiracy of such magnitude that it could potentially rank as one of the most sinister in history. The result of this conspiracy is that millions of people are living unhealthy lives and dying prematurely. Serious diseases such as diabetes, heart disease, cancer and Alzheimer's have increased dramatically in the last fifty years. By far the most obvious consequence of the conspiracy is that so many people are now overweight. As a society we have almost come to accept this as inevitable, but it is not. The conspiracy is perpetrated by the food industry and supported by the major food advisory bodies. Thankfully, we are able to tell you how you can easily transcend the misinformation and get your health back on track.

The epidemic of obesity and associated diseases is a modern phenomenon which we are led to believe is due to leading a more sedentary lifestyle and eating fatty foods. This is simply not true. The conspiracy gets deeper when the so-called solution to obesity is to eat more of the very foods which are causing the problem in the first place. In years to come, we believe the current mainstream health advice will be viewed as one of the biggest mistakes in nutritional history.

The culprit for all these problems is simply the consumption of more and more refined carbohydrates, and the relentless pressure to do so. We are told by the health authorities to cut down on fat and to eat more carbohydrates. Whilst carbohydrates are not inherently bad, the modern Western diet contains far more refined carbohydrates than the body evolved to eat. Sugar,

1

refined white flour and corn syrup are amongst the products which the body simply cannot deal with in the volumes we consume them. Once you realise this, supermarket shelves will never look the same again. You will see the rubbish we are being encouraged to eat is everywhere and the misinformation is totally pervasive.

As supported by much research, when the modern Western diet reaches an indigenous population you can start a stopwatch. Within twenty years, diabetes, heart disease and cancer rates will soar. Terrible consequences ensue, including amputations of limbs, blindness and early death. We have no intention of telling the full and tragic story in this little book – more details can be found in *Why We Get Fat* by Gary Taubes, and there are many other good books out there (see Appendix D).

This little book was conceived as a result of a Facebook page Richard Leach ran called *Cut The Bullshit: Truthful Nutrition and Fitness Advice*. As Richard's friend, Justin Whittaker decided to try the diet which Richard was writing about. To be honest, at this point Justin was cynical about Richard's dietary philosophy. Much to his surprise, Justin ended up losing over twenty kilograms of unwanted fat and immediately realised the truth of Richard's writings. This led Justin to also research how it could be that the nutritional advice he had been brought up with could be so wrong. He arrived at exactly the same truth as Richard. Both Richard and Justin are passionate about spreading this truth.

This book is a collection of 100 tips which we think will help anyone improve their health and fitness. The central theme is a low-carbohydrate lifestyle. We will begin with some basic information about how to get started on a low-carb diet. If you want an in-depth discussion on the biology of low-carb living, perhaps start with some of the excellent books out there on the subject and come back here for valuable health tips. If you are on the fence and not sure if low-carb will work for you, why not give it a go, if only for a week, to see what happens? Scepticism is not a barrier to weight loss on this diet!

The evidence for low-carb eating is now overwhelming and we do not intend to add to that. The diet Richard follows is the Slow-carb Diet (SCD) developed by Tim Ferriss and presented in his book *The Four Hour Body*, but this is just the diet that Richard has found to be most effective – we are fans of most other low-carb eating plans, for example, Paleo, or the low-carb diet developed by Robert Atkins (before the brand name was sold). It is up to you to find the one that suits you best. Justin's weight loss was based on counting the carbs he ate each day to ensure he stayed 'low-carb', but Richard simply ate low-carb foods without the hassle of keeping count. Both approaches work fine. They ultimately achieve the same thing.

The first five tips tell you what you need to know to get started on your low-carb diet. Subsequent tips are pretty much in random order, although we do refer to previous or later tips where necessary.

We suggest you read a tip a day and try to put the suggestions into practice over a period of time. You don't need to follow every tip, but the more you can do the better. Also, if you already have a good fitness regime, you can ignore the fitness tips and just concentrate on the diet tips.

Note that in this book we refer to 'weight' when we actually mean 'mass'. Strictly speaking we should not talk of weight in units of kilograms, but everyone does, so we have here. Richard, being a physicist, insisted on this note!

OK, let's get started…

Tip 1: Get your doctor on side

Each and every human body is different. You may have pre-existing health issues which make switching to a low-carb diet unadvisable. We are not health professionals so our very first tip must be to advise you to talk to your doctor.

In 99.9% of cases, your doctor will be delighted that you have decided to lose weight – which is universally accepted as being a healthy choice. We advise you to ask your doctor for a 'fasting blood lipid test' before you start the diet. This will tell you, amongst other things, the state of your good and bad cholesterol levels (see Tip 53). These figures will be a useful starting point for you and your doctor to see trends as your low-carb diet progresses.

In nearly all cases your doctor will be able to show you that your cholesterol levels and triglycerides have improved dramatically as you follow the low-carb diet. You will also note other benefits, such as a lower blood pressure, which all reduce your risk of heart problems.

Obviously, if your doctor advises against following a low-carb diet or if you are pregnant, then do not proceed. We cannot recommend you put your child on a diet of any kind. By all means we encourage you to cut down on the sugary, refined foods you give them, and offer healthier choices. But dieting and children is not an area which has had much research and we are not in a position to recommend it.

Tip 2: Decide on your target weight

If you are overweight it is a good idea to set yourself a target weight. Be ambitious. Set a target which is slim and healthy for your height. To work out your ideal weight for your height, use a Body Mass Index (BMI) calculator, which can be found on the internet, for example at:
http://www.nhs.uk/Tools/Pages/Healthyweightcalculator.aspx
This will tell you the weight to aim for within the 'healthy weight' range and to take you out of the overweight or obese range.

Note that there are issues with using BMI as a health indicator but in this context, i.e. setting your target weight, it is fine.

Tip 3: Keep a calendar of your weight-loss progress

Before you start your diet, measure your weight and write it on a calendar. Each week, on the morning of the same day (for example, every Saturday) write down your new weight. Do not weigh yourself every day. Your body's mechanism for water retention is not exact, and you will drive yourself crazy with odd drops and gains if you weigh yourself too often. However, you should see a definite downward trend week on week.

Usually in the first week you will lose the most – a few kilograms – but much of this will be due to water loss. After this you can expect, on average, to lose half to one kilogram of fat a week. Keep your target weight in mind and look forward to the day you will, almost inevitably, reach that weight. You will have a sense of achievement as you look back on your progress, as your weight slowly and surely drops, bringing you so many benefits in way of health, mobility, fitness and self-esteem.

If you really want, you could also track vital measurements such as your percentage fat (see Tip 20) or dimensions around the stomach line or thighs.

Tip 4: Be prepared for the doubters

Do not be put off doing a low-carb diet because of the doubts of other people. To put it simply – just do it! Within the first week you will see that it works. And each and every week that you lose weight will confirm that you are doing the right thing.

There will be many who are very vocal that you should be eating low-fat food and the foods we will be advising you to avoid. We are used to following the advice of professionals and food agencies, but you will see for yourself that, in this case, they have got it very wrong. Rest assured, there is much published scientific evidence supporting low-carb weight loss.

Tip 5: Get into fat-burning mode!

Here we get to the crux of losing weight on a low-carb diet. Your body can run in two power 'modes'. It can burn glucose (from carbohydrate) for energy, or it can burn fat (which it gets from your fat cells). Your body comes ready-made to run in these two modes – evolution is a wonderful thing. However, with the modern diet, we tend to be running almost exclusively in glucose mode.

Here is the simple key to losing weight, and it really is this simple: switch to fat-burning mode. This is done by limiting the amounts of carbohydrates you consume, so your body is forced to burn the fat stored on and in your own body. This does not, by the way, involve you going hungry at all. Nor does it put your body under any stress, it is entirely natural. You will still be eating healthy, filling food. But at the same time, your body will be burning your own fat as a by-product, as the human body has evolved to do.

So now you know – it is called a low-carbohydrate diet because we limit our intake of carbohydrates so we can naturally burn fat. By the way, when you reach your target weight you can stop the severe reduction in carbohydrate intake, but we'll cover this later.

Tip 6: What is carbohydrate anyway?

The content of the food we eat contains fat, protein and carbohydrate in varying proportions. The body converts certain types of carbohydrate into glucose which it burns as energy. Some carbohydrate is in the form of fibre, which is not digested but assists in the passage of food through our intestines. Fibre is a good thing.

In general, naturally occurring sources of carbohydrate, such as vegetables, fruits and grains, come along with many beneficial micro-nutrients which are important for health. But in the modern Western diet, these nutrients are stripped away to form what we call 'refined carbohydrates', which are doubly bad in that they are converted to glucose far too quickly, causing many health issues which we elaborate on later.

In order to lose the excess fat you have gained through eating refined carbohydrate, you will temporarily restrict the carbohydrates you eat. If you are concerned that you may be missing out on nutrients during weight loss, simply take a good quality vitamin and mineral supplement daily. We also think this is a good idea even after you have lost weight (see Tip 36).

Tip 7: What to eat to lose body fat?

Firstly, let's just come out and say it: fat as a food source is not a bad thing. Yes, every label you have ever seen saying 'low fat' is misleading you to believe this is the healthy option. Dietary fat has been demonised since you were born (unless you are way over seventy years). Secondly, eating fat does not make you fat. Indigenous Greenlanders eat a huge amount of fat and blubber, and are neither overweight nor suffer from heart disease or diabetes at anything like the rate of the rest of the world.

Actually, body fat is the result of the excess of glucose in your blood being turned into fat and getting locked into your cells (see Tip 18 for more details). And this glucose comes primarily from carbohydrate. So, from now on, don't recoil when you read about eating fat. Any doubts you have about eating fat will be dispelled within the first few weeks as the fat on your body, counterintuitively, drops off.

There is one very important exception to the fat rule. This is trans-fats. These really are very unhealthy man-made fats and must be avoided. More about these in Tip 73.

In simple terms, what you do on a low-carb diet is cut down on the amount of carbohydrate you eat, and increase the amount of protein and fat to compensate. You will not be counting calories. However, to begin with, you may very well have no idea how much carbohydrate different foods contain, so how are you to cut down?

There are two approaches, and you can choose which one suits you. If you are a free spirit and want to pick and choose what to eat and drink from all the foodstuffs, you need to know exactly how much carbohydrate foods contain. Or you can simply follow religiously the 'what to eat' tips which follow, and not bother counting.

For those who want to count carbs and come up with their own ideas of what to eat, refer to Appendix A, which lists the amount of carbs in food and drinks. If a food is not listed, a search on the internet will always turn up an answer. For example, search for 'carbs in white bread' and you'll get your answer.

If you are going down the carb-counting route, a good rule-of-thumb to lose weight is to not exceed 35 net carbs per day (see Tip 67 on how to calculate net carbs). At this level, you will almost certainly be in fat-burning mode. Bear in mind that this restricted level is only for the weight-loss phase. When you reach your target weight you will be able to increase the level of carbohydrates (this is covered in Tip 50). Seeing as refined carbohydrates were responsible for you getting fat in the first place, you will be well advised to introduce only natural, non-refined carbohydrates so you don't put the weight back on again. These may be in the form of whole grains and nutritionally dense vegetables.

The tips which immediately follow go into more detail about the food you should be eating and what you should be avoiding.

Tip 8: Breakfast

For many first-time low-carbers (if they are trying to lose body fat), breakfast can seem a little daunting. Cereals are out, as is toast. So what's left?

For convenience, there are a couple of low-carb breads available. In the UK there is 'Hi-Lo' bread and 'Liv-Life' bread. These are also very high in protein which helps block the absorption of the carbohydrates they contain. Large supermarkets stock these brands; just search online for your nearest stockist. A couple of slices of these low-carb breads toasted, along with plenty of butter (not margarine) and perhaps some almond nut butter, marmite, or unsweetened peanut butter will set you up for the day. Or toasted with a couple of eggs on top are good too (fried, scrambled, poached – up to you). But do avoid conventional bread, both white and brown; it is very high in carbohydrates.

A good old English fry-up is also allowed. This will put a huge beam on some people's faces, but is just too heavy and hard work for others. You also don't really want to eat processed meats every day as they can contain nitrites as preservatives. If you can source organic bacon and sausages without nitrites, so much the better. You can eat as many eggs as you like and even boil them the night before (don't worry about the egg/cholesterol horror stories – see Tip 60). It's good to get some fibre if you can - any salad or veg will do (Richard likes spinach as it's ultra-healthy). A few legumes will also help to keep you energised until lunch-time.

On weekdays, try two fried eggs, a handful of lentils (from the tin) and a little pile of spinach (cooked from frozen). This takes well under five minutes to cook. At the weekends, try egg, bacon, tomatoes, mushrooms, spinach and the occasional sausage. There are hundreds of alternatives which can be found with a little internet searching, although many of them are not acceptable if you are following the Slow-carb Diet, and some of them are a bit dubious on any low-carb diet (if you are trying to lose body fat).

It is important to eat breakfast within one hour of waking (within ½ hour is better – this ensures your body's metabolism fires up appropriately and has been shown to have a significant effect on weight loss) and always have some protein. If you really can't handle protein sources, such as meat or eggs, take a low-carbohydrate protein shake. This factor alone can mean the difference between steady weight loss and none at all.

Tip 9: What can I eat?

This tip is assuming you want to lose body fat - if not, you can be more relaxed – see Tip 50 on maintenance. You want to keep your body in fat-burning mode, which means keeping your blood sugar low. Firstly, the foods listed below are going to be low in carbohydrates. Secondly, foods can be ranked according to their 'Glycaemic Index' (GI). GI is a measure of how quickly the carbohydrate is turned into glucose and, therefore, how likely your insulin is going to be activated, causing fat storage. Basically, you want to avoid anything that is going to cause insulin spiking – that is, anything with a GI greater than or equal to about 30 (see Tip 27).

Read the back of products and keep the carbs low. It is difficult to give an exact figure, but the lower the better if you want to lose fat – you don't 'need' any. Stay below 35 net carbs per day for rapid weight loss. You will probably still lose weight on 60 net carbs a day, but start 35 as a sure-fire way to kick-start the process.

These lists are not exhaustive – you need to do your own research. But here's the basics:

1. All meat products, but watch for hidden breadcrumbs in sausages, and you should try to eat good quality meat and minimise processed meat where possible.
2. Any seafood – the more the better – avoid breaded fish.
3. Eggs – as many as you want.
4. Most green veg and salad, plus cauliflower
5. Most legumes.
6. Dairy, including cheese – most low-carb diets allow dairy so long as it is full-fat. Justin ate cheese and dairy during his weight loss and continues to do so.
7. Fruit – the best is low GI fruit, for example most berries, but keep it to a minimum. Some low-carb diets do not allow fruit as it is high in fructose (see Tip 58).
8. Fat – see Tip 63 on fats, but animal fats and butter are great, olive oil and nut oil are good, vegetable oil should be avoided. Don't be scared to eat the fat and skin on meat.

Things to avoid include: anything with sugar, pasta, rice, potatoes and other starchy veg, bread and all cereals.

To drink you can have water, tea or coffee. That's about it – avoid all sodas and especially avoid fruit juices.

We'll cover booze later, but it's not brilliant news if you like a good tipple! Spirits are generally acceptable neat or with zero-calorie mixers. But bear in mind that fat loss will stall while your body burns off alcohol. This will just slow down your fat loss a little.

Never eat anything that says 'low fat' or 'low calorie'. To get them low they have to use all sorts of chemical tricks and add loads of junk. Plus the fat is often the only good part, so why the hell get rid of it?

Tip 10: What to drink?

If you are trying to lose body fat on a low-carb diet, the simple answer to this question is: water, tea and coffee. Nothing else. You should be drinking a lot of water anyway. Water is very important to your health and helps you flush out all that body fat (fat leaves the body primarily through your pee and breath).

The best form of tea is green tea, preferably leaf not bag – Richard drinks about ten to fifteen cups a day (see Tip 25). Drinking coffee is fine, so long as it is not full with sugary additives. You can use full-fat cream or milk in some low-carb diets but not the Slow-carb Diet (no dairy). Too much coffee is bad for other reasons, but you know if you have too much!

Tim Ferriss recommends Yerba Mate tea, especially to help you poo on a binge day (see Tip 69). Fruit juice is a definite no-no; you may as well just drink sugar-water.

Tip 11: Vegetable oil

We have been told for years by our nutritionists that vegetable oils are good for us because, according to them, unsaturated fats are much healthier than saturated fats. On the contrary, they can be very bad for us and contribute to several diseases. The same holds for seed oils, for example, soybean oil, sunflower oil, corn oil, canola oil, cottonseed oil, safflower oil, etc. And, we can lump margarine in with this lot. This advice does not apply to plant oils such as olive oil, coconut oil and most nut oils (although it is better to try to keep the cooking temperature as low as possible).

The way the harmful oils are made/processed would make your toes curl, but many of the points below apply whatever method is employed. Here are some reasons why they are so unhealthy:

1. They contain very large amounts of biologically active fats called omega-6 polyunsaturated fatty acids, which are harmful in excess.

2. Omega-6 and omega-3 fatty acids are biologically active and humans need to eat them in a certain balance to function optimally. Excess omega-6s in our cell membranes are prone to harmful chain reactions.

3. Certain essential molecules made from omega-6 and omega-3 fats are crucial in regulating inflammation in the body. The more omega-6s you eat, the more systemic inflammation you will have. Inflammation can contribute to various serious diseases, including

cardiovascular disease, arthritis, depression and even cancer.

4. They contain a large degree of trans-fats (see Tip 73).
5. There is evidence from both randomised controlled trials and observational studies that vegetable oils can increase the risk of cardiovascular disease.
6. Their consumption is associated with various other diseases and issues, for example, increased omega-6 in breast milk was associated with asthma and eczema in young children and a correlation between the consumption of these oils and homicide rates in the USA.

Bottom line: don't touch any of these oils, ever.

Tip 12: Eat enough

Sometimes when people have tried other diets, and due to the brainwashing given out by most health folk and nutritionists, people think they should be restricting how much they eat. THIS IS NOT THE CASE WITH LOW-CARB DIETS. You should eat at least three meals a day, and eat enough to fill you up and last until the next meal.

Sometimes you may need the odd snack in-between, but we'll come on to snacks in other tips. Of course, be sensible – i.e. don't eat for the hell of eating; eat to fill you up. This is an essential tip. If you do not eat enough, you will not promote fat burning. Despite saying that, if you want to, or have to, skip a meal sometimes (once a week or so), that's fine, so long as it's not breakfast. Don't skip breakfast (except the day after a binge day – see Tip 42).

Nuts do not fill you up and they are packed with calories. So one handful of nuts a day is all you should be eating.

Tip 13: Eating with the family

If your partner doesn't want to follow you on a low-carb diet then what to do? It is perhaps a worry that you will have to be cooking two meals each time you eat. In actual fact, you will find that all of the foods you will be eating are delicious and not weird or cranky at all.

For those who still want their carbs, just include portions alongside what you are cooking for yourself. For example, if you are having a meat stew with vegetables and cauliflower rice, just serve the same stew to your partner but substitute the cauliflower rice for normal rice or pasta. Or, if having fish, serve your partner with potatoes, but have extra portions of vegetables for yourself.

Tip 14: What is a beer belly?

There is a belief that the paunch that men get in middle age (sometimes called a beer belly) is caused by the stomach stretching due to drinking or eating too much. It may be considered no cause for concern because the measurement at the waistline, where the belt sits, is quite normal.

The truth of the beer belly is far more sinister, however. In actual fact, what appears to be a stretched stomach is the result of the accumulation of fat around the internal organs. This is called visceral fat and is a major indicator of impending heart problems. Thankfully, this fat is one of the first fats that is burned for energy when you follow a low-carb diet. You are almost certainly adding years to your life by losing your beer belly, and have the benefit of feeling years younger with a flat stomach.

Tip 15: To binge or not to binge?

When we talk about binging in this book we are talking about temporarily breaking all the rules and eating whatever you want for one day a week. No foods are off limits.

Why would you want to do this, given that we have written this book about how carbs are clearly the enemy?

If you are severely overweight, a low-carb diet will be a slow and steady route to losing weight. There is some evidence that, if your body loses weight for a prolonged period of time, your metabolism may slow down. This is a natural response, which is meant to avoid starvation and may stop weight loss in its tracks. Binging once a week will trick your system into not thinking it is steadily losing weight. Note that there are also good hormone-based reasons for binging (see Tips 81 to 84).

If you only have a few kilos to lose, it is unlikely you will physically 'need' a binge day. But if psychologically it will help you stick to the plan then by all means go for it. Also, if you make this a weekend day, it allows you to go out with friends and family and eat exactly the same as them.

Both Richard and Justin can attest to the fact that eating carbs one day a week does not stop you losing weight. You will gain weight that will take a couple of days to shift, but if you stick to only getting on the scales once a week – before binge day – you will see that you are losing steadily. In actual fact, this weight gain is mainly water which gets bound to the glycogen that is stored in your body as fuel.

Justin found binge day interesting in that it really highlighted his addiction to certain carbs. Chips (French fries) were his weakness and the more he ate the more he wanted to eat. Nowadays Justin rarely eats chips as he clearly has issues with them, and he likes to feel in control.

Even when you have achieved your target weight, you have choices. Some will carry on eating low-carb during the week, and continue with a binge day at the weekend.

Others will gradually increase daily consumption of healthy carbs with no need to binge.

Some low-carb diets encourage a binge day, and some forbid it – the choice is ultimately yours. You may find, as many do, that your desire for refined carbs diminishes over time. Or you may find that you can't live with the thought of not eating the forbidden foods at least once a week. Either way, your health will be so much better when you have attained and maintained a slimmer you.

Tip 16: How to binge effectively

If you decide to have a binge day, then the best advice is simply to 'go for it'. Try to have a normal, low-carb breakfast, but after that you can eat as much of whatever you want, including all the banned foods.

Our ancestors were perfectly adapted to binging. They would have long periods of not eating and then gorge on whatever they could get their hands on. And we are still the same – having a blow-out will not harm you (within certain limits of course).

There should be no restrictions in terms of amount on binge day. In fact, it is better for you to fill up good and proper – this will kick your hormones in the right direction (see Tips 81 to 84).

There are a host of techniques that can be followed to try to reduce any weight gain due a binge day (See Tip 42). Do try to have a normal, high-protein breakfast though and don't start on the sweet stuff until after this.

Tip 17: Initial effects of low-carb

A friend of ours recently attempted to go low-carb but had some nasty side-effects. He felt tired, low, with some muscle soreness and food cravings. This is basically a 'come down' effect of sugar addiction. Sugars (i.e. carbohydrates) affect the same parts of the brain as recreational drugs and are highly addictive (see Tip 24). When you stop 'using' them, there may be a short adjustment period. Some people don't even notice this, most people have a low day or two, but for some it can last for up to a week (very rare).

The physical effects will not stop you going about your daily activities, so our advice is just put up with it; it will stop. The cravings will also reduce as you break the addiction, but you need to keto-adapt before that happens. Keto-adaptation is when your body switches from using glycogen (sugar, i.e. carbs) as its energy source and starts using stored body fat (see Tip 43). This will only occur if you are strict about not eating carbs – if you continually screw up, you will simply prolong the agony. Carbs also float around in the blood stream (as your blood sugar) and retain water. So, when you stop eating carbs, you will see a relatively large reduction in weight (up to 3 kg) in the first ten days or so. This is usually a point when everyone gets elated and thinks the diet is amazing; it's the reason many other diets seem successful when trials are run over short periods. All of the effects are basically your body adjusting to its natural way of eating – the way we evolved to eat. As soon as you are keto-adapted, you should start shedding 0.5 to 1 kg per week, and that will be body fat, not water.

So, if you are thinking of starting low-carb, be prepared for a short period of adjustment and, if it's a little tough, just remind yourself that the end result is losing all your unwanted body fat, increased energy, improved concentration, better sleep and better skin condition.

Tip 18: Fat loss explained in more detail

There is only one way to lose body fat and that is through a process called lipolysis. Lipolysis is the body's natural process of breaking down fat to make energy. This requires specific biological conditions. But first, there are three ways of producing energy:

1. Glycolysis – this is the breakdown of carbs in the form of starch and sugars. Glucose is the product, and this is fed into what's called the Krebs cycle to produce energy via breathing.
2. Lipolysis – this is the breakdown of lipids in the form of oils and fats. The result is ketones, which are also fed into the Krebs cycle via the same route.
3. Protein synthesis – this is a last resort method and is covered in Tip 52.

The switch between glycolysis and lipolysis is controlled by hormones and dictated by complex feedback mechanisms that inform cells when to produce energy.

Glycolysis in an anabolic (body-building) state, which is controlled by insulin – the hormone that regulates blood sugar (or should do). When insulin is in control, we are growing – muscles, tissues and fat stores. Insulin is produced when we eat carbs; it promotes glycolysis and inhibits lipolysis. Therefore, fats you eat during glycolysis cannot be used for energy and are locked away in fat cells, making them difficult to release. Excess carbs are stored, first as glycogen, then as fat. Gaining weight is always a result of glycolysis and always involves insulin.

Lipolysis is a catabolic (body-breakdown) state, which can only occur in the absence of insulin. During lipolysis, the fats you eat, and have stored, can be used for energy. Lipolysis can occur only when all the carbs we have eaten or the glycogen we have stored is used up. All weight loss is a result of lipolysis.

Again, eat carbs = make insulin = burn carbs, not fat. Carbs run out = insulin levels fall = burn fat.

We should switch easily between glycolysis and lipolysis according to the food we eat and our energy stores. The effect on our fat stores means we always gain a little bit of weight after meals then lose a little bit before the next meal. Hunger and fat storage should be regulated so that we end with neither a gain nor a loss (homeostasis). But, overweight bodies don't work efficiently. Homeostasis is disrupted and for unknown reasons, some of us make too much insulin, so that when we've burned all the carbs, there is still some insulin left. This causes insulin resistance. The excess circulating insulin inhibits lipolysis and we can't get to the fat even though we've got no carbs. This results in a lack of energy and a feeling of hunger. When this happens for a prolonged period, we go into long-term storage mode and pack away the fat. The only way to break the cycle is to stop overproduction of insulin: lay off the carbs.

When insulin resistant folk try to lose weight by reducing calories, they go round and round experiencing low energy, low motivation and hunger. They can lose weight by starving themselves, but this is dangerous and ineffective

It is not overeating and lack of exercise that leads to fat storage. It's lack of energy and hunger that lead to overeating! This is a physiological disorder, not a psychological one. All you need to do is restrict carbs, and the problem goes away. So, there you have it in a nutshell. You just need to restrict carbs for a period, then slowly start introducing them, i.e. follow a low-carb diet. Bingo.

Tip 19: Dieting is a fantasy

It always amazes us how many people think that they can follow some diet, lose a load of weight, then stay that way when they go back to eating 'normally'. The common experience is that people in fact gain weight, and this is perfectly understandable. So, don't do that!

You have to realise that you need to find a way of living that is sustainable. Yes, you can use techniques to get your body fat (not necessarily your weight) down and then try to maintain that level (your 'set point' – not so low that everyone tells you that you look too thin), but going back to old habits of eating badly, is just not going to work. This seems totally obvious to us, but has created the entire diet industry – an industry able to function on the desperation of so many people and bad advice given out by governments.

So, you need to find what works for you and make that your life. If you don't think you can stick to it, you probably won't. Personally, we find low-carb eating easy and enjoyable and it improves our lives. The option of a binge day means you don't really have to give anything up. Plus low-carb is infinitely more appealing than the usual starvation diets. But you need to prove this to yourself.

Note that the infamous Weight Watchers is pretty much now a low-carb diet – in fact, many of them are heading in that direction. That said, most of the 'big' diet regimes are steeped in fantasy, so beware and stay away from them. So, don't diet; change your life, forever!

Tip 20: Measuring body fat

On a ketogenic (low-carb) diet you will lose body fat. On a low fat/low calorie (starvation) diet you will lose body fat but also muscle.

How can you monitor exactly how much body fat you are shedding? Apart from booking yourself into specialist flotation tank facilities (this is by far the most accurate technique), there are two easy methods.

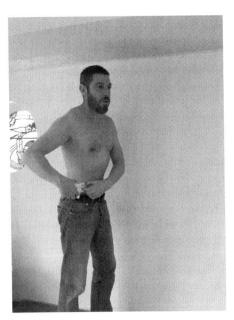

1. Use pinch callipers – these can be bought online for less than £10, are easy to use and can be relatively accurate (see action shot).

2. Use bathroom scales that have a body fat sensor (actually measures electrical resistance).

Electronic devices are not accurate but they

will show you trends (up, down or plateau). We have both and they agree within about 1% of each other and follow the same trends, until you get to about 13% body fat, then the pinch callipers become the most reliable.

It is very important to take a measurement at the same time after waking up and before you put anything in your system. Only have one weigh-in a week, and make it the morning of your regular binge day (if you have one). Your weight will vary a great deal over the week, because of the binge, but more on that in later tips.

As a professor of metrology, Richard would suggest taking the average of three measurements each time. The scales will give you readings of body fat percentage and visceral fat percentage. Note that by far the best way to see whether you have lost body fat is to look in the mirror. If the scales or callipers say you are going up or down but you can clearly see otherwise, don't believe them.

Tip 21: Fitness goals

Lots of people find it hard to get, or continue to be, motivated for exercise. That's because we are basically not meant to exercise for no reason. Whilst getting in shape and feeling better are reason enough for some, many folk need an extra push.

One of the best ways to keep you motivated is to have a goal. But this goal really needs to be something tangible. Simply getting fitter or losing weight are not enough motivation for most people. Achieving a particular personal best time or distance for an event may be enough, but it is easy to let things slip. So why not sign up for something, for example a run, a cycle ride, swim, walking holiday, skiing, etc.? Actually putting something in the diary and writing out a training schedule really helps to keep you motivated. And once you have done it, have a rest, then sign up for something else. There are countless events available on the internet and many of them are local. You can also do something for charity – that really helps with motivation.

Richard recently did a mud run and is currently coming to the end of a sixteen-week weight-training challenge. The mud run forced him to go from not-having-run for several months to a decent 10k pace in a few weeks – there is no way he would have done that unless he had the event lined up. Next on the horizon is a 100-mile bike ride – from scratch. Motivation depends on a lot of factors, but if you put something in the diary, it will help you to keep focus.

As a side note, Justin, with his inquisitive nature, deliberately did not take exercise while testing out the low-carb weight loss approach. He wanted to know, categorically, that the weight he lost was due to the change in the food he was eating. He simply carried on walking his dog once a day as he had always done. He lost almost 20 kg, no problem. Don't take this as the way to go though, this was done just through curiosity.

Tip 22: Is exercise good for weight loss?

We have been told for years that exercise is an excellent way to lose weight. It seems almost sacrilege to dispute this. But it is not so – exercise is not an effective way to lose weight.

Now, we have to be careful here – everyone should follow a well-planned exercise regime and the benefits are immense. There is some evidence that, if you do not exercise, it is equivalent to smoking: you will get ill more often and die earlier. But exercise is not an effective way to lose weight.

If you do the simple mathematics and work out how much exercise you have to do to burn calories, it is quite shocking. A 10k run will burn about 800 kcals – that's a fairly decent meal. All you do is burn off what you just ate. Also, remember that if you are not keto-adapted (following a low-carb diet), then the first thing you will use to power your exercise is your glycogen store, and this is approximately 2000 kcals.

Plus it's just not as simple as calories in calories out. Whether you use fat as your energy source (and therefore burn it) will depend on your current fitness level, how much you rest, what you did the day before, what you eat, etc. If you are well-rested, it is possible to burn as much on a one-hour walk as it is on a one-hour run.

Lastly, when you do lose weight using cardiovascular exercise, it will be fat and muscle that goes. Obviously, if you do enough exercise, you will lose weight – over-weight marathon runners are rare. But we've all seen people who spend hours in the gym but are still overweight.

Research seems to indicate that 80% of your weight loss should be down to diet. Richard's motto is 'diet for weight loss, exercise for a fuller life'. It is essential to do both, but if weight loss is your goal, concentrate your effort on getting your diet right and exercise for fun.

Tip 23: Cardio

Cardiovascular (CV) or aerobic exercise is any exercise involving relatively low intensity, usually repetitive action. It includes running, walking, swimming, rowing, cycling and work on the cross-trainer. It is not interval training or resistance training. Some say that it should not involve anything above 85% effort, as this leads to anaerobic exercise.

The big question is: how much should you do? The answer to this question will vary a great deal depending on your fitness goals, but we suggest you do not use it to try and lose body fat, at least not as the primary part of your weight-loss armoury.

The benefits of a good CV routine include:

1. Reducing the risk of heart disease and stroke – such conditions are the biggest causes of illness and premature death in the UK, and probably the rest of the world (not forgetting the effects of smoking).
2. Reducing high blood pressure, which leads to the same cardiovascular benefits as point 1.
3. Promoting healthy blood sugar levels, therefore, reducing the risk of type 2 diabetes and other illnesses in many organs of the body.

4. Improving levels of 'good' cholesterol, therefore reducing the risk of heart disease.
5. Reducing joint problems and lower back pain, for example osteoarthritis and osteoporosis.
6. Improving your immune response; helping you fight all sorts of bugs.
7. Reducing the risk of certain cancers.
8. Making you feel good – not to be understated.

If you just want to keep fit and healthy, our suggestion is broadly in line with that of fitness author Mark Sisson. You should do one (max two) resistance sessions (see Tip 66), one session where you go to 100% a few times (see Tip 99) and two to five hours of 'easy CV' at less than 85% effort.

The 'easy CV' can be anything you like, including daily activities and playtime. That's it! Any more than this, unless you are training specifically for a sport activity, can be counter-productive. Richard goes out running, cycling or walking – two to five hours soon adds up. Walk or cycle to work and you'll eat up loads of your allowance.

It is a really good idea to have a training session for how to run, or at least look up some techniques on the internet. Just going out and running is okay, but may lead to injury. Richard had a knee operation caused by running and, when he got a specialist to check his style, he had been running badly for years. Just a single training session is probably all you need (plus some effort to put the new style into practice).

Tip 24: Sugar – is it toxic?

Table sugar, or sucrose, consists of approximately 50% glucose and 50% fructose.

One problem with excessive amounts of sugar is to do with the fructose. Fructose, unlike glucose, can only be processed by the liver. If we overload the liver with sugar, the fructose gets turned into fat, and some of it lodges in the liver. This process can lead to fatty liver disease.

The liver should contain no fat. When it does it can lead to inflammation and scarring. If this continues for a long period, the liver could stop functioning.

There are other arguments to suggest that excessive sugar is toxic. Excessive glucose in the blood is extremely toxic, and this is normally handled naturally by the body with the release of insulin. But consistently high levels of insulin can make cells resistant to it. The end result is metabolic syndrome, obesity, heart disease and type II diabetes. Many scientists believe that having constantly elevated insulin levels can cause cancer.

For some, sugar is addictive, in the full biological meaning of the word. Like drugs, reward chemicals are released when we consume sugar. For those with addictive tendencies it is probably wise to avoid sugar.

And don't think you will be missing out nutritionally if you cut down on sugar. It contains literally zero essential nutrients. The calories from sugar are called 'empty calories' for this reason.

Tip 25: Green tea

Green tea is made from unfermented leaves that are pale in colour and slightly bitter in flavour, produced mainly in China and Japan. It has also turning out to be somewhat of a 'super food'. Many East Asian folk drink green tea, hot or cold, all day long and it is purported to be one of the contributors to the long lifespans enjoyed by many of them.

You can pretty much drink green tea in place of water, although it does contain caffeine, so you do need to be a little careful. Often, the amount to make one cup can be topped up with water many times; reducing the amount of caffeine per cup.

Make sure you get a good brand if possible – loose leaf is better than bags. You can buy bags to fill up nowadays, if you can't handle using loose leaf varieties.

Here are some of the benefits – and there is evidence behind all of them, they are not just hearsay:

1. Green tea contains various bioactive compounds that can improve health – it contains various nutrients, antioxidants and some minerals. Some of these have health benefits and are probably what has led to the anti-aging reports.

2. It improves brain function. This is primarily an effect due to the caffeine, which has been intensively studied and consistently leads to improvements in various aspects of brain function, including improved mood, vigilance, reaction time and memory. But green tea also has amino acids, which (especially when combined with caffeine) can relieve anxiety. Note that green tea has much less caffeine than coffee and produces a very different 'buzz'.

3. It affects fat burning and improves physical ability (it increases metabolic rate). There are many studies which show these affects for green tea.

4. The antioxidants can decrease the chances of contracting various types of cancer.

5. The bioactive compounds in green tea can have various protective effects on neurons and may reduce

the risk of both Alzheimer's and Parkinson's, the two most common neurodegenerative disorders.

6. The catechins in green tea may inhibit the growth of bacteria and some viruses. This can lower the risk of infections and lead to improvements in dental health, a lower risk of caries and reduced bad breath.

7. Some controlled trials show that green tea can cause mild reductions in blood sugar levels. It may also lower the risk of developing type II diabetes in the long term.

8. Green tea has been shown to lower LDL cholesterol, as well as protect the LDL particles from oxidation. Observational studies show that green tea drinkers have a lower risk of cardiovascular disease.

What isn't on that list is that green tea is delicious. As with most such drinks, it takes a little getting used to, but it is well worth the switch.

Tip 26: Is dietary fat fattening?

Not as much as we have been led to believe. In the 1970s, some really badly reported science made a link between dietary fat and obesity. Basically, twenty-two countries were surveyed and only the seven that showed a positive correlation were reported (even though the others showed no, and even negative, correlations). Without naming names, this spurred on the rubbish we are told about dietary fat making us fat. Now, there are ways that the body can turn dietary fat into stored fat, but it is not the usual route.

If you use carbs as your primary fuel source, then too much dietary fat can be converted into sugars, which are then converted back to fat for storage. But most will be excreted.

If you follow a low-carb diet and, therefore, you use fat as your primary energy source, then virtually all dietary fat will either be used as fuel or excreted (unless you swallow a whole bottle of oil or something silly like that). So, if you are following a low-carb diet, you have nothing to worry about dietary fat (except getting enough).

You can eat butter, lard, skin and fat on meat, and many oils (but avoid all vegetable or seed oils). Exactly what types of fat are good and bad will be covered in a subsequent tip, but stay well away from trans-fats (see Tip 73).

Tip 27: The Glycaemic Index (GI)

The GI is a measure of how quickly the amount of glucose in your blood (blood sugar level) rises after eating a food type. Glucose has a GI of 100 and all other food is referenced to this. The closer a food type is to 100, the more your blood sugar will increase when you eat it, therefore, producing insulin and the more likely you are to store fat. This is all somewhat simplified, as this is a complex process, but as a good rule of thumb is that if you stick to food low down the GI scale, you are less likely to store fat.

Some example foods: starchy potato, white rice and most cereals are high GI and should definitely be avoided; some other potatoes, most breads and a Mars bar are moderate; and fruit, veg and legumes are relatively low. The numbers vary a little depending on where you look, so watch out. Meat is zero GI. Table sugar is about 60, so not as bad as potatoes or cereal, but it is poisonous in many other ways (see Tip 24).

The glycaemic load is a version of GI that takes into account portion sizes, which obviously have an effect. For low-carb dieting, you need to stick to low GI foods. See Appendix B for a list of food types and their associated GI. More detailed lists can be found on the internet.

Tip 28: Water

As discussed, when talking about what you can and can't drink, you should (and need to) drink plenty of water when low-carb eating, especially if you want to lose body fat.

On average, the quantity of water in an adult body could fill 45 litre bottles. Why so much water? Because water is absolutely critical to life. In fact, most cells in the human body are composed of more than 75% water. Without it, none of them would be able to function.

A good rule of thumb for how much water to have each day, is about nine glasses, plus one extra for every 10 kg overweight you are. If you're finding yourself stuck on a diet plateau (see Tip 39), look at your water intake. Of course, you need even more water if it's hot or if you're exercising vigorously.

Water has several vital functions in the body. It:

1. Delivers to each cell the nutrients needed to carry on the processes of life.
2. Dissolves vitamins, minerals, amino acids, glucose and other nutrients.
3. Provides a medium for chemical reactions.
4. Is involved in the production of energy.
5. Lubricates joints.
6. Acts as a shock absorber inside the eyes, spinal cord and joints.
7. Helps the body flush out waste materials.
8. Helps maintain the body's temperature.

So, get drinking, even if you have to pee more often. When producing ketones, pee is one of the main ways that body fat exits – you are literally peeing your fat away! Note also, that if you drink green tea, that counts towards your water intake (but watch the caffeine).

Consider getting a water filter of some sort. If you don't have an under-counter filter, a filter jug is just as good. It improves the taste and removes chlorine, lead and bacterial contaminants.

Tip 29: Dairy

Many low-carb diets allow unlimited consumption of dairy products, so long as they are full-fat varieties. So you can eat cheese, milk, cream, butter and yogurt until the cows come home (sorry).

However, there are some things to bear in mind. The problem with low-fat varieties is that they have usually had all sorts of nasty processes applied to extract the fat (why?), they often have additives to give them flavour and they can be fairly high in carbs. So check the labels to make sure the food is full.

The Slow-carb Diet does not allow dairy (except on the binge day of course). This is because there are sugars in dairy (lactose) and these can spike some people's insulin levels, leading to fat storage. The SCD does allow butter, though, and encourages the use of it for frying.

If you seem to be having trouble losing fat, perhaps cut dairy out if you can, then slowly introduce it back in when in maintenance. As with all potentially insulinemic foods, you need to find your insulin tolerance. This should be a slow and patient process of trial and error.

Tip 30: Warming up

It is essential to warm up before doing any exercise, aerobic (CV) or anaerobic (resistance or high intensity). Warming up should not be avoided simply because it is the less exciting part of exercise. Warming up increases muscle speed and economy of movement by getting blood and hence oxygen running though the muscles. It also allows the heart rate to get to a workable rate for the subsequent exercise and gets you mentally focused.

Warming up can be as simple as a five-minute slow jog or cycle, but will depend on what exercise you are doing. If you intend to do anything strenuous, dynamic stretching is the best (those funny movements you see footballers doing before they play).

We can't advise you on what to do for every exercise, so take expert advice on this one. Note that warming up should not be done via static stretching – this can actually be damaging, so save it for after your exercise.

Tip 31: Warming down

Warming down after exercise is essential for a number of reasons. It aids in the dissipation of waste products (for example, lactic acid) and allows the heart rate to return to its resting rate. Warming down can be as simple as a five-minute slow jog, but will depend on what exercise you are doing, so take expert advice.

Tip 32: Post-exercise stretching

Whilst stretching may seem a little boring, it is essential if you want to avoid unnecessary soreness and injury. Before exercising, you should be doing dynamic stretching – static stretching can actually be counter-productive. Stretching after exercise has the following benefits:

1. Reduced muscle tension.
2. Increased range of movement in the joints.
3. Enhanced muscular coordination.
4. Increased circulation of the blood to various parts of the body.
5. Increased energy levels (resulting from increased circulation).

Stretching becomes increasingly necessary as we get older. We can't suggest what stretches to do; that is highly dependent on what exercise you do, so you'll have to ask your trainer or do some research. Also, how long you stretch each muscle group will depend on your goals. Up to about ten seconds is the minimum amount to stretch and thirty seconds and over is becoming progressive. Yoga moves are an excellent way to stretch. So, however boring stretching may be, get it done.

Tip 33: Vegetables

We thought we should stress the importance of having vegetables as part of a low-carb diet. Not only are vegetables high in fibre (see Tip 40) and loaded with vitamins and minerals, they contain myriads of substances called phytonutrients or phytochemicals. These compounds are probably the explanation for why people whose diets are high in vegetables are at a lower risk for cancer, heart disease, certain eye conditions, and many other health problems.

Phytonutrients can act as antioxidants, boost our immune systems, repair cellular damage, and much more. There are hundreds, perhaps thousands, of these compounds – impossible to obtain through supplement pills. Some low-carb diets say to cut veg at the beginning. We say, do not follow this advice. Your fat loss may be a little slowed, but this is much better than missing out on so many benefits.

A large proportion of almost every meal, including breakfast if possible, should contain veg (probably more than half the portion). You should of course be avoiding starchy veg (for example, potatoes, swede, beets) if you want to lose body fat, but you can look up the GI of veg and keep it low (see Appendix B). Carrots are OK in moderation. A good rule of thumb is that you should only eat a lot of veg that grows above the ground.

Tip 34: Low-carb desserts

Many desserts are off-limits as they contain sugar – one of the purest forms of carbohydrate there is. But there are a few desserts we find are very satisfying and totally allowed.

Our favourite dessert would be a type of fresh berry, either blueberry, strawberry or raspberry. Add a big spoonful of cream – either clotted, crème fraiche, double cream or ricotta cheese.

We sometimes like to add a spoonful of ground flaxseed, and maybe a few pine nuts. Justin eats a bowl of berries with cream practically every day.

Sprinkle with a little powdered Splenda to sweeten if required.

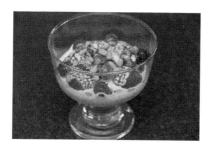

You can also use almond flour (or ground almonds) and coconut flour to bake with. There is an example of a low-carb chocolate cookie in Appendix C. Also, if you search the internet for low-carb desserts, or diabetic desserts you will find many recipes using these flours.

Artificial sweeteners are always used in place of sugar. We find liquid sucralose is the best tasting, with powdered Splenda coming second. Liquid sucralose is available online and has less carbs than Splenda. Splenda does have carbs in the powder, but weight for weight it is much less carb dense than sugar.

Tip 35: Vitamin C

Vitamin C (ascorbic acid) is one of the best known vitamins. We all know the stories of sailors suffering with scurvy and bleeding gums due to the lack of this essential vitamin. But vitamin C has many more health-giving properties.

The recommended daily amount is 60 mg. This amount was set long ago, and is really the minimum needed to prevent scurvy. Humans and primates are amongst the few species which have lost their ability to manufacture vitamin C. It is, therefore, essential to our health. Amongst the other animals which can synthesise vitamin C, the amount per kilogram is far higher than the human recommended daily amount. Amounts of more than 60 mg are perfectly safe and 500-1000 mg daily supplements are available in supermarkets. The only known side effect of very high doses is diarrhoea, but this varies from person to person.

Vitamin C is found in many fruits that are often restricted whilst on a low-carbohydrate diet, the most obvious being oranges. A good quality multivitamin will make up for deficiencies, but the best source is food. For low-carbohydrate sources, there is broccoli and other dark green vegetables, red peppers, blackcurrants, strawberries, tomatoes, and lemon juice. Be aware that cooking and storing food depletes the vitamin C content considerably.

Vitamin C is used rapidly by the body so if you take a supplement, consider spreading the dose throughout the day.

Here are just a few health benefits of vitamin C:

1. A powerful antioxidant which helps to protect cells and keep them healthy.
2. Helps fight infection. Antibodies and white blood cells lose vitamin C during illness.
3. Helps prevent LDL cholesterol from oxidising and forming plaques in the arteries.
4. Helps cope with stress by supporting the adrenal gland to manufacture anti-stress hormones.
5. Helps facilitate wound healing.

Tip 36: Supplements

We recommend a high-quality combined vitamin and mineral supplement. But remember that supplements are just that – something that is used to supplement a lack of something else. If you had an excellent diet, you wouldn't need to supplement at all. That said, most people can't eat oily fish four to five times per week, don't get enough sunlight, don't eat enough protein and so on. Intensive farming methods have depleted the soils of many trace minerals. The minerals are essential to the creation of crucial enzymes that your body needs.

Don't buy cheapo supplements! Don't get the supermarket brand. Have a look around and get a well-reviewed brand (most brands are available on Amazon and have good reviews), even if it costs you a few more pennies.

Justin takes Solgar VM2000 Multinutrient every day. Richard takes a multi-vitamin and mineral (Sanatagen A-Z Complete), a vitamin D and an omega-3.

Tip 37: Constipation

One of the potential side-effects of a low-carb diet is constipation. The problem can be caused by a combination of the changing biology of your dietary system and/or a lack of fibre.

Constipation is easily cured; try one or a number of the following:

1. Drink more water (you should be doing that anyway).
2. Eat more fibre, especially veg.
3. Take probiotics.
4. Increase the amount of salt in your diet.
5. Take a fibre supplement. Psyllium husks are available in supplement form and work a treat.
6. Try taking a magnesium supplement.
7. Try flax oil.
8. Yerba Mate tea is recommended by Tim Ferriss and green tea is a wonder drink.
9. Exercise can also help.

The only thing we would advise against is constantly taking laxatives; whatever kind. Laxatives will relieve the symptom, not get to the cause. A good source of fibre is much better for you.

Of course, you may have a medical issue, so if things persist, see a doctor.

Tip 38: Legumes

A legume is a simple, dry fruit contained within a case or a pod. The most well-known legumes are peas, beans, peanuts and lentils. Legumes have a somewhat high GI (see Appendix B), so many low-carb diets do not allow them (for example, Paleo: no, Slow-carb Diet: yes). It is best to stick to specific diets during weight-loss periods – the 'inventers' of the diets have usually put the ground work in and know what combinations work best. But in the maintenance phase you can experiment with legumes. Here are some of the purported health benefits of consuming legumes:

1. Legumes are high in protein and fibre.
2. Legumes provide a steady source of glucose for energy – they may be high GI, but they release carbs very slowly (often called slow-release carbs), so insulin is not necessarily spiked.
3. Legumes are high in folate and iron, and have appreciable amounts of magnesium, manganese, copper, selenium, molybdenum, and antioxidants – all good chemicals – in varying amounts depending on the legume variety.
4. Legumes are associated with reduced risk of colon cancer – the jury is still out on this one, but it could turn out to be a big plus point for legumes.

And, just to be balanced, here's the potential negative sides:

1. Legumes are hard to digest and, hence, make you fart more!

2. Legumes can aggravate auto-immune diseases – the jury's out on this.
3. Legumes are high in starch and carbohydrates.
4. Legumes contain estrogen mimics, which can be harmful to health – the jury's out on this but we wouldn't give children soy beans.
5. Legumes can shrink your brain – very weak evidence for this.

So, a mixed bag of beans (sorry). Our advice: stick to your diet rules for weight loss, then mix it up and see what happens.

Tip 39: Plateaux

On any weight loss regime, you will eventually hit a plateau. After the wonderful steady loss in weight, it suddenly stops, despite not changing any aspect of the diet. This could be because you have hit your natural minimum, but it is more likely to be a 'weight loss plateau'. This can be caused by a number of factors, for example:

1. Not eating breakfast soon enough after waking up – try to eat breakfast within an hour of waking, even half an hour if possible. And, of course, make sure you are eating enough protein for breakfast (see Tip 8). If you really can't handle eating protein, take a shake.
2. Not eating enough protein (see Tip 52).
3. Not drinking enough water (see Tip 28). You should be drinking water like it's your job. The only valid replacement is green tea.

4. Your hormones are telling you to hold onto your fat reserves – the best way round this is a binge day!
5. Not eating enough (see Tip 12). Yep, not eating enough can quite easily cause you to keep the fat, contrary to what we have been told for decades.

There are a host of ways to break a plateau, for example: the reverse of the above (you can take a protein shake on waking to address two of them), changing your exercise routine and even eating more. But, usually the best cure is patience.

Last time Richard took the journey down to his natural minimum (i.e., the point at which it is not possible to lose weight without resorting to extreme measures), he hit a plateau of around 14% body fat. He was there for five weeks and tried all of the above methods to break it. He doesn't know if one actually worked, but it just went away and he went quite rapidly down to his natural minimum of 11%.

So, when it happens (and it probably will happen), we suggest you just stick with the programme and start taking action if it is still not broken after six weeks. Plateauing, and even multiple plateaux during the descent, is normal, so don't give up in desperation!

Tip 40: Fibre

Fibre is present in all fruits, vegetables and grains. It is a carbohydrate, but it passes straight through us with no chemical interaction, so it does not raise your insulin levels (and, therefore, cause fat storage). Fibre is one of the essential parts of a diet (including protein, fat, and vitamins and minerals), and its role is to prevent sugars in food from being digested too quickly, and to ease the passage of food through your system.

So, when you calculate the amount of carbs (if you are restricting them during the first stage of some low-carb diets), you need to subtract the amount of fibre from the total carb count. In the US food will display total carbs and fibre, so what is called your net carbs is the difference. That's the count you should use. In the UK and EU, only digestible carbs are shown on food labels, so you do **NOT** deduct fibre. (see Tip 67).

Note that low-carb diets get a rap for resulting in constipation, but this will not necessarily be the case so long as you keep your fibre level high (see Tip 37). So, fill up with veg and think about getting some psyllium husks.

Also, beware the misinformation about breakfast cereals being good sources of fibre. They are generally packed full of bad carbs (and usually a load of other rubbish), so don't use this as your fibre source. Our advice on breakfast cereals: avoid them all!

Tip 41: Atherosclerosis – the truth

Heart disease and heart attacks shorten the lifespan of millions of people every year. The incident rate of coronary heart disease has soared in the last century. It is a disease that was almost unknown before the modern high carbohydrate diet became the norm. It has now earned the dubious title of number one killer of Americans.

Atherosclerosis is a condition where vital arteries to the heart become narrowed by plaque. This restricts the blood flow to the heart and can stop it working properly. If the plaque ruptures, a clot can be formed. This can cause a heart attack or interfere with blood supply to the brain, causing a stroke.

Excessive insulin (produced by eating large amounts of refined carbohydrates) is strongly indicated in the formation of this arterial plaque. A low-carb diet inherently reduces the amount of insulin being produced, reduces bad LDL cholesterol and hence reduces the risks of arterial plaque and heart disease.

Atherosclerosis certainly goes hand-in-hand with obesity. When you lose weight, and keep the weight off, the danger of atherosclerosis and heart disease diminishes substantially. This applies no matter what diet you follow. We happen to believe a low-carb lifestyle is the easiest way to lose weight and keep it off. You really will increase your chances of living longer by losing that excess weight. Keep this in mind as a strong motivator if you get a craving for junk food: it is literally going to kill you!

Tip 42: Minimising the effects of binge day

The inclusion of a binge day into a low-carb diet has a two-fold purpose:

1. It has a psychological effect in stopping us thinking we're missing out on anything (this may be important to you for sustainability).
2. It stops the metabolism from down-regulating (thinking it is starving).

You will always weigh a few kilograms more after binge day – this is due to more water being absorbed by the carbs you've eaten. You should lose the extra weight in a few days and definitely by the next binge day (one week or so). But, what you actually want is either all the nasty carbs to pass straight through you or all the glycogen to go into your muscle tissue and not get stored as fat.

Tim Ferriss recommends a number of tactics for reducing fat gain during and after binge day and these can be found on his web site.

The really simple ones are to have a normal breakfast with plenty of protein, a squirt lemon or lime juice on all your meals (this reduces insulin production) and down a pint of grapefruit juice before your first high-carb meal (this tells your liver to get ready for the onslaught). Richard also drinks Yerba Mate tea (see Tip 69) with each meal and consumes vast amounts of green tea as always. Oh, and drink even more water than normal on binge day.

Another way to minimise the fat gain effect, and to get you back to ketosis faster, is to skip breakfast (and preferably lunch) the following day. This should be relatively easy as you'll be stuffed full of glycogen. You may like to burn off the glycogen in the morning with a serious resistance session (or interval training), then fast until evening dinner. Even better to go for a long walk also, but only if you're pretty fit. Lastly, burning off your glycogen store the night before a binge day is also a good idea. Happy binging folks!

Tip 43: Ketosis

After a short period of being on a low-carb diet (from a couple of days to a couple of weeks), you should go into ketosis. The level of carbs to reach this state is something you need to find by experiment, but most good low-carb diets will teach you about this process.

Ketosis is where your body switches from using glycogen (from carbs) as its primary energy source, to using fat. As you reach ketosis (or near ketosis) you will start to control insulin production. It is the production of insulin that causes the body to store fat and keep it in storage. Ketones are the by-product of the fat burning process, and they are excreted via your pee, skin and breath (you literally pass fat).

Ketosis is not to be confused with the state that diabetics can get to where they produce large amounts of ketones. This state is known as ketoacidosis and is caused by a dangerous lack of insulin – see Tip 98). Ketoacidosis can have various physiological effects.

As you become ketogenic, you should get an increase in energy and become more clear-headed. You will also not get such extreme hunger pangs when you go without food. If you want to test for ketones, you can buy ketosticks (from for example Amazon) which you pee onto and observe the colour change.

Some say that ketosis is a secondary process as a defence against starvation. We think it is *the* primary process, as it would have been the natural state for our ancestors for hundreds of thousands of years. Despite reports to the contrary, ketosis is not a potentially dangerous state. Many civilizations have been ketogenic, for example Inuits, American Indians and Masai. Few are now because they met us and ruined their perfectly healthy diets by introducing grains and sugar (and alcohol).

Tip 44: Low-carb and blood sugar

Having a stable blood sugar level is a major benefit of sticking with a low-carb diet. When you eat refined carbs, your blood is immediately flooded with sugar. Your body has to do something about this quickly as high concentrations of sugar are poisonous. This is dealt with by the secretion of insulin, which transports the sugar into your cells. You will often experience general lethargy, irritability and food cravings after this brief spike and drop in blood sugar.

Over time, with a constant barrage of sugar and insulin, your cells may become resistant to insulin's effects. The body copes with this by producing even more insulin. Then a downward spiral of health begins until it gets to the stage where you may become diabetic.

As the headlines attest, there has been a dramatic increase in diabetes since the 1980s, when the high-carb diet was first touted as the healthy option. It has often been called an epidemic, and we wouldn't disagree with this.

On a low-carb diet you will have stable blood sugar throughout the day. You will, therefore, have more energy and experience fewer food cravings. Dietary fat has no influence on blood sugar whatsoever and protein, when eaten with fat, has only a moderate effect that is not unhealthy.

Tip 45: Rest

Sufficient rest is an essential part of any fitness regimen. As anyone who has got seriously into fitness knows, exercise can be very addictive. As long as it doesn't start to deleteriously affect your life, such an addiction is not a bad thing. But sometimes this addictive tendency can get in the way of the necessary balance between exercise and rest.

If you are training for a particular sport activity, then you can let the balance slip for short periods of time. But, even high-level athletes have periods of high-intensity training and off-season periods of rest. If you are not training for a sports activity but just want to be fit and healthy, then there is no excuse (or reason) to not rest enough.

Rest will allow muscle growth, fat burning (yes, if you are ketogenic and suitably trained, you can burn fat whilst sleeping) and repair. How can you work to your best if your poor body is constantly repairing itself and you have a permanently low immune system?

We can only give loose advice on rest as it will depend on what you want to achieve and your physiology, but we would say you should be doing no more than one to two interval sessions a week (including spinning) and no more than two to five hours of easy CV. If you're doing resistance, one to three times a week is ample, and you should not exercise a muscle if it is still aching from the last time.

Exercise should make you feel more energetic throughout your life. If it seems to make you less energetic, then you are doing too much. You'll also pick up injuries if you overdo it.

Every now and then, you should have an extended rest period for a week (up to a month). It will not do you any harm at all. You'll know when you are getting the balance right because you will be injury free and feel good. So if you want to be fit and healthy, remember the chill pill is as important as the hard stuff.

Tip 46: Travelling

Low-carb diets can be a bit of an issue when on the move. As soon as you get to airports or train stations you are in a high-carb zone – surrounded by sandwiches, rolls and crisps. Of course, if you can get to a restaurant, you're usually fine (the Giraffes at Heathrow are more than happy to cater for you), but most of the meal deals and snacks, in the likes of Boots or WHSmith, are high-carb.

The best thing to do is to think ahead and take your own food, but this is not always possible. When you are in this situation, its often nuts that come to your rescue, and you can allow yourself to have a little more than the 'good handful', as you're not having anything else. Pork scratchings are another tasty snack along with Peperami or cooked chicken. Salads are OK, but watch the hidden carbs in the dressings, croutons and other extras. Most in-flight food is no good, so it's a good idea to time your binge day if you are doing long haul.

Another alternative is to go without and use the time as an excuse for a mini-fast. You won't do yourself any harm, and now you are keto-adapted your blood sugar shouldn't drop too low.

Richard travels a lot, so has worked out all sorts of coping strategies and knows the airport food shops inside out. Probably the best solution is to eat plenty before you leave and take your own food with you.

Justin will take a packet of macadamia nuts with him if he thinks getting decent food may be an issue. This tides him over until proper food is available, and macadamia nuts are delicious so it's no hardship.

Tip 47: Nuts

All low-carb regimens (except Atkins for the first two weeks) allow nuts to be eaten. This is good and bad news. The main problem is that people start using nuts as a snack. So, what's the problem? Well, in case you hadn't noticed, nuts do not fill you up (well not unless you eat buckets full). In fact in Richard's case they just make him hungrier and want to eat more nuts. Richard can easily eat a whole big bag of roasted cashews (and does allow himself the pleasure on binge day).

The rule of thumb is: one good handful of nuts a day, no more. Richard finds its best not to have them in the house! The problem is that, whilst we are not counting calories in low-carb diets, nuts have massive amounts of stored energy and are the exception to the rule. So, try to keep it to a handful a day or you will stall fat loss.

Note that peanuts are legumes, not nuts, so if your low-carb regimen doesn't allow legumes, don't eat them. Note also that nuts do vary in their low-carb content (see Appendix A) – almonds and macadamias are best and cashews are worst, but stick to a handful a day and you can probably get away with any type. Sweet-coated nuts are out, for example honey roasted and check the label for carbs on other coatings.

Tip 48: Low-carb flour

Normal refined flour is a complete no-no when living a low-carb lifestyle. White or wholegrain flour is very high in carbs as are all foods made from them. There are several low-carb versions of flour which can be used for baking. Which one you choose will depend on:

1. How low you need to keep your carb count.
2. What sort of baking you need to do, i.e. what texture and consistency.

All the substitutes have some carbs, so we would just stay away when losing fat, but you can definitely use them during maintenance. Note also that these substitutes are not cheap, so probably just for treats. The main versions are:

Almond flour – finely ground almonds. Good source of fat and fibre, but it won't rise. Great for cakes and biscuits.
Soy flour – some people don't like the taste of this and it won't rise.

Whey powder – not the best substitute as the texture is not quite right.

Flax seed meal – great substitute, high in fibre and very high in omega-3.

Coconut flour – tasty but results can be quite dry.

Lastly, you can use some grain flours but they are relatively high in carbs, so make sure to read the label.

Tip 49: How low should I go?

Some people wonder when they should stop losing weight or if they can get down to dangerously low levels of body fat. If you use a low-carb regimen to strip body fat (along with some exercise), you will eventually plateau at a healthy level. The weight loss will simply stop. You may even see a gain if you do any resistance training and gain muscle.

To go lower, you would have to use extreme dieting methods or very high levels of exercise. So, you have nothing to worry about. You can either stop when you are happy with your mass and/or fat percentage or carry on until you plateau. It is highly likely you will hit a false plateau before the real minimum (see Tip 39).

Note that if you use starvation (i.e. low-cal/low-fat dieting) to lose weight, you will lose muscle and fat, and it is possible to lose too much. However, this is extremely rare and most people simply won't have the willpower or stamina to starve themselves for so long. Conclusion: use a low-carb method and you'll get there in a healthy way.

Tip 50: Maintenance

After successfully losing body fat on a low-carb diet, you will probably be very happy with yourself, and rightly so. Big pat on back. Once you are happy that you are low enough, you can start maintaining, as opposed to losing.

It is easy to begin adding small amounts of carbs back into your diet. Some people seem to do it as a reward for successfully losing weight, others do it subconsciously. Either way, continuously cheating on your diet will increase carb cravings and eventually cause fat gain. Dieting should be thought of more as a lifestyle change, or else it could result in a vicious cycle of weight gain that becomes tough to break.

So, the way to do it is to try one type of carb, for example, some fruit after exercise or porridge for breakfast. Do it for a week or two and see if you gain. But, mixing and matching here and there in an uncontrolled manner will probably result in disaster. Get control of your life and slowly see what you can get away with. Or just stay low-carb – with a binge day, this should be enough for anyone.

As we've said, we are of the belief that refined carbohydrates are not good for you. By in large avoid them, seeking out non-refined versions wherever possible.

Tip 51: Omega-3

Omega-3 fatty acids are essential – we cannot make them ourselves in our bodies, so we have to take them as part of our diet. Omega-3 fatty acids come in a variety of forms, but the most essential ones are DHA and EPA. The best food to provide this is fish, but if you don't eat enough fish you should take a supplement.

Supplements come in a variety of forms, but the best one is fish oil. Many of the vegetarian varieties do not contain enough DHA and EPA, so the veggies need to read the labels and shop around.

Studies show that taking omega-3 can help lower triglycerides and blood pressure, and even help with things like depression. There were some scare stories recently about the dangers of omega-3, but the real issue is with the additives put in cheap supplements, not the omega-3 itself. It is well worth spending a little money on good supplements – never buy the cheapest varieties.

Ground flax seed can be sprinkled onto many foods and is a rich natural source of omega-3 and other healthy minerals.

In conclusion, omega-3 fatty acids are essential and you must get them from somewhere. The best way is to eat loads of fish, but if you don't, then take a good supplement daily.

Note that omega-3 supplements should be stored in the fridge (or at least in a cupboard away from sunlight), as they can oxidise and spoil if left out.

Tip 52: Protein

How much protein should we eat each day? Protein is one of the essential parts of our diet. It is the primary source of material to repair and build almost all parts of our body.

Contrary to popular belief, low-carb diets are not (or should not be) high-protein diets. They are 'right-amount-of-protein' diets. Exactly how much protein you should be taking in is difficult to calculate and will depend on your dimensions, weight, age and exercise goals. But try to get around 20 g per meal. You can find grams per day values for your specific diet, but there are a few simple rules.

You should try to eat protein at every meal, including breakfast (Tim Ferriss suggests you should be trying to get 40% of your daily protein at breakfast to decrease carb impulses, so get those eggs in).

You don't need to eat meat to get protein, but it is the easiest source and packed with so much goodness. Unflavoured whey protein is the best substitute if, for example, you can't face eggs and meat at breakfast.

If you are trying to gain muscle and need to have a certain amount of protein a day, there is no evidence that you can't have the bulk of it in one sitting, i.e. you don't need to spread your intake through the day.

Taking a protein shake within twenty minutes of finishing anaerobic exercise (resistance or intervals) is common practice and is reputed to help reduce muscle soreness and aid the repair process. Evidence for the effectiveness of this is scant but many do it anyway.

Note that a lack of protein can also lead to a weight loss plateau (see Tip 39).

Tip 53: Cholesterol

The 'C' word is often banded around when people are running out of ammunition with which to attack low-carb diets. 'But surely cholesterol will increase due to all that saturated extra fat?' Well, total cholesterol may, but here's the important story.

There are basically two types of cholesterol. LDL is the 'bad' stuff that brings increased risk of heart disease as it gets deposited in cells, especially artery walls, where it can cause plaque build-up and blockages. HDL is the 'good' stuff, which is collected from cells, taken to the liver and excreted via bile. So high HDL means you are getting rid of it and is good news. Also, 20% to 30% of our cholesterol comes from food, and the rest we make ourselves.

Cholesterol is related to the amount of carbohydrates you eat (actually to the level of insulin required to deal with them). When insulin increases, our bodies go into fat-storage mode, by converting excess glucose to triglycerides and causing the liver to produce cholesterol. These triglycerides then travel around the body and are stored in fat cells. It is at this point that the LDL is also deposited in to artery walls.

When insulin levels go down, glycogen (a hormone which works in balance with insulin) is produced. Where insulin stores nutrients, glycogen breaks them down for energy. When glycogen takes over, fat is broken down for energy (it is this process which releases excess water, resulting in rapid weight loss at the start of any diet). So, when you low-carb diet, your total cholesterol may increase, but the LDL will go down.

It is very difficult for doctors to measure the difference in cholesterol types, so you often just get a total reading and everyone jumps around saying that your new diet is killing you. This is rubbish. Low-carb dieting is much better for you in terms of cholesterol levels (as well as every other health indicator we know of).

To put his money where his mouth is, Justin recently went to have his cholesterol tested via a fasting blood test. The results were, according to his doctor, 'absolutely top class – whatever you are doing keep on doing it'. LDL cholesterol was very low, and HDL was high (a good thing). Justin was expecting this result, but it is nice to be reassured. We'd highly recommend you do it too – it's fun to wave the results in the nay-sayers' faces!

Tip 54: Cramps

Some people experience cramps when they go low-carb, especially if you also increase your exercise level. As you keto-adapt, the tasks of your liver change somewhat and you tend to release more salts, for example sodium, potassium and magnesium. Also, you are probably eating less packaged food, so you will eat a lot less salt. And, you should be drinking more water and peeing more often. A deficit of salts can cause cramps, often in the calf at night, which is highly painful.

Many people suggest taking supplements to replace the lost salts, but often the cure is simply to have a ¼ teaspoon of salt a day. You can get this by just having the salt, using more salt in your cooking or drinking a stock cube.

Note that all hunter/gatherer (therefore, ketogenic diet) civilizations (for example Inuit, American Indian, Masai) had ways of getting salt into their diet, for example using sea water or drinking blood. You can try the latter if you want, but otherwise, a little pinch of salt is usually all you need. We happen to love salt, so no problem here.

Tip 55: Muscle soreness

A short time after resistance training, high-intensity interval training and the like (anaerobic exercise), you may get muscle soreness. It takes typically from 24 to 48 hours to kick in, depending on your fitness levels and how often you train. But, can you do anything to prevent it?

Short answer: not a lot.

Long answer: there are a few tricks to help, some coming from personal experience, some from hearsay. Some say that taking a mix of protein and carbs straight after a session can help, but we are clearly not going to encourage you to take carbs! Richard takes a whey protein shake within twenty minutes, but has no idea whether this stops soreness or not.

Stretching should always follow any exercise, and Richard is convinced this helps (he does seem to hurt more if he doesn't). Cycling for a couple of minutes after leg resistance work also helps. Supplements can be used (L-glutamate is an obvious one), but you need to experiment.

There are also more professional minimisation methods such as direct icing (frozen peas are good here), alternating hot and cold showers and 'eccentric reps' (look it up if you are interested).

Many like muscle soreness as it tells them they are getting somewhere and it's rarely that bad. If you are resistance training and you are not getting any muscle soreness, then you probably are not getting gains. We would suggest you need to tweak your routine – keep the body guessing.

Another question is: should you exercise that muscle when it is sore? Again the jury is out: some say you should fully rest the muscle before working it again, others that waiting for soreness to fully subside is the best way to maximise the chance of getting sore again. So, a mixed bag of advice. You'll have to experiment, and we would be keen to hear your stories and findings.

Tip 56: Peas and sweetcorn

Peas are fairly starchy as vegetables go, so people on low-carb diets don't usually eat a lot of them. Still, peas are not nearly as starchy as potatoes or sweetcorn and are a rich source of nutrients, so fitting them in from time to time is a good thing, if it works for your particular diet.

½ cup peas = 7 grams effective (net) carbohydrate plus 4 grams fibre and 59 calories. ½ cup frozen uncooked peas = 7 grams effective (net) carbohydrate plus 3 grams fibre and 55 calories. The average GI of peas is 48.

Sweetcorn is usually thought of as a vegetable, but it is probably more accurately categorised as a grain (and, indeed, is sometimes called a 'whole grain'). A corn plant is essentially a grass with exceptionally large leaves and seeds. Given this, it should be no surprise that corn is high in carbohydrates, mainly starch.

½ cup raw corn kernels = 18 grams effective (net) carbs plus 3 grams fibre and 89 calories, ½ cup canned/frozen corn kernels = 14 grams effective (net) carbohydrate plus 2 grams fibre and 67 calories. An average GI of 54 is commonly used, but varies a lot from this value (up and down).

You may wish to avoid both unless it's binge day. There are plenty of other vegetables to choose from.

Tip 57: Feeling tired?

People feel tired for all sorts of reasons, and sometimes blame it on a low-carb diet. The fact is that you should have *more* energy on a low-carb diet than a high-carb diet, so if you are feeling tired, you are not doing it properly or it's something else. We are not medical doctors so can only give some pointers here based on experience. Here is a list of things you should look at if you are feeling tired:

1. Are you getting enough exercise? We'd recommend at least one sprint session, one resistance session and two to five hours of easy CV (walking, running, cycling, etc.) per week. You can get away with skipping the sprinting and resistance sessions without affecting your energy levels (but will miss out on a whole host of other benefits).

2. Are you exercising too much? Loads of folk we know do far too much high-intensity CV (for example, three or more spin sessions a week). If you feel lethargic, have aching muscles and a bit moody, take a break. When you exercise, you also need to rest (see Tip 45). We'd say, unless you are training for something specific, stick to the amount of exercise in 1. Also, take a week off from time to time – you won't lose anything.

3. Are you eating enough? You should be eating until you are full up and not feeling hungry (see Tip 12).

4. Are you sleeping enough? How much will vary on the individual, but we all know when we don't get enough.

5. Are you stressed, worried or have other such issues? This can massively affect how you feel. If you are, take positive steps to do something about it.

6. There may be a specific part of your diet that is missing, for example not enough protein or fat, so look at your diet's advice and tick off what you should be getting.

7. Are you boozing too much or taking other drugs? We'll leave that one to you to work out.

8. Do you smoke? If you do, concentrate all your effort on stopping – it is the most stupid thing you have ever done, and will kill you and generally ruin your shortened life.

9. Are you drinking too much caffeine?

10. Are you drinking enough water (see Tip 28)?

Of course, there may be a short period of increased tiredness as you keto-adapt (see Tip 17), but just remember, you should feel better on a low-carb diet, not worse.

Tip 58: Fruit

Should you eat fruit on a low-carb diet? Some low-carb diets allow small amounts of fruit (for example, Paleo) and some do not (for example, Slow-carb Diet). Fruit has a dual personality. On the one hand it is packed with good vitamins, minerals and fibre. On the other hand, it is high in sugars and will, therefore, spike your insulin and cause fat storage. It is definitely not as bad as it would seem just by reading its GI. Some fruits are particularly high in sugar (for example, bananas and apples) and should be avoided when losing weight. Dried fruits should also be avoided.

Berries, such as strawberries, blueberries, blackberries and raspberries, are okay to eat in small amounts as they are low in carbs. They are also packed with healthy antioxidants.

When trying to lose weight (fat), don't eat fruit apart from perhaps a small amount of berries. When you are happy with your weight, introduce fruit slowly and see if you start gaining or not.

Whatever you do, do not drink fruit juice – you may as well just eat out of the sugar bowl!

Tip 59: Sandwiches

Pretty much the main snack at lunchtime in the UK is the 'great British' sandwich. So what happens if you can't eat bread? There are many alternatives and you can also get some good low-carb breads in the main shops these days (see Tip 87).

When at work, you could take in leftovers from the night before. When travelling, simply find something else. Most big stations or airports have somewhere where you can get a packet of salad and some cooked chicken. Or you can fall back on nuts, but watch the amount (see Tip

47). Also, many use this as an opportunity to fat – they can skip a meal and feel almost no effect.

When you are in the situation where there are only sandwiches, for example, the classic business lunch (especially in Germany), simply wait until others have finished then take the filling out. You might get some funny looks, but who cares? We do like a packet of pork scratchings too, but control the amount again.

Tip 60: Are too many eggs unhealthy?

Short answer: no, not at all. The fear of cholesterol rising with egg consumption is completely unfounded. The body produces its own cholesterol (see Tip 53). If additional cholesterol is added by eating eggs, the body adjusts its own production level to keep it almost constant (unless you have some illness which affects this process).

Eggs are a great source of protein, plus vitamins and minerals, and have fat-burning properties. The following website is packed with information about the health benefits of eggs. Interesting to note the bit at the end about scrambled eggs: they are best eaten without being smashed up.

Richard eats a minimum of two eggs every morning and uses boiled eggs as snacks. They are basically a super-food, so start eating them regularly especially for breakfast.

Check out:

http://health.howstuffworks.com/wellness/food-nutrition/facts/health-benefits-of-eggs.htm

Tip 61: Glycogen store

Even if you are keto-adapted (following a low-carb diet), you will still have a store of sugar (glycogen) which is used as a sort of immediate energy source, and is integral to muscle growth. This will come from the complex carbs you are eating (veg, legumes) and from protein synthesis.

So, if you really want to be efficient at burning fat, do some high-intensity activity (for example, some serious lifting or interval training), then go for a nice long walk. You will deplete your store and then burn purely fat. It's also a good idea to burn off your store before and after a binge day.

This is one of the reasons why interval training is so effective: it can leave you burning off pure fat for days. This is also why long sessions of cardio (called chronic cardio) is so ineffective: you are simply burning off your store.

Tip 62: Low-carb alternatives

There are plenty of branded 'low-carb' foods you can get these days. Our advice: be wary. Unfortunately, this industry has been infiltrated by the same folk that make low-fat/low-calorie products. They use every trick in the book to get the apparent carb count down and you just can't trust what you're eating.

Stick to real food, prepare and cook it yourself and have a vague idea of where it's come from. Especially avoid low-carb energy bars or anything that has 'sports' written on it. As mentioned before, we have found some low-carb breads to be good, for example Liv-Life and Hi-Lo brands.

Tip 63: Fats and oils

There are various types of oils that are an essential part of the food we eat and are known in their most basic components as fatty acids. These are hydrocarbon chains with a bit of oxygen at the end (the 'acid part'), but are not generally classified as carbohydrates (which have a lot more oxygen in them). They are essential to our diet, including the 'saturated' fats (SFAs) that in recent decades have been labelled as unhealthy. Most of this has now been discredited and it is unlikely that SFAs have any significant detrimental effects on our health; they are in fact an important part of our diet, and have very important roles in our cells.

We can separate fats into two basic types: saturated and (poly)unsaturated. Saturated means there are no double bonds between carbon atoms. Unsaturated means there are some double bonds and polyunsaturated means there are more than one of these in the molecular chain.

Unsaturated oils can be further separated into other types, of which there are three that are commonly encountered in food: omega-3, omega-6 and omega-9. The omega number represents the position of the first double bond from the end of the chain.

In general, one might hear that unsaturated oils are better than saturated ones. This is not true; they both have their uses in the body. In the case of unsaturated oils, generally omega-6 oils constitute a much larger proportion of our diet than omega-3 (particularly in Western diets), and the balance between the two is important – because of the excess of omega-6 it is important to get as much omega-3 into our diet as possible. Omega-6 oils are not intrinsically bad in themselves, but they compete with omega-3 and the ratio needs to be kept stable. An imbalance in ratio can affect LDL/HDL cholesterol ratio, which contributes to the build up of plaque in arteries.

A good source of omega-3 is oily fish such as salmon and mackerel, or flax seed for vegetarians, although flax seed is not as beneficial because the omega-3 oil type is different (see below). For vegetarians who need to supplement this essential ingredient, there are algae sources available. Vegetarians must also be careful to take certain other supplements such as vitamin D, iron and vitamin B12 which is generally lacking in plant matter, but some of which is available in dairy products for non-vegans.

Omega-3 comes in several types. All are essential because the human body cannot make them from other oils. The basic vegetable source is alpha-linoleic acid (ALA). This has some benefits but is limited. More complex types found in fish and algae are EPA and DHA. These can be made from ALA in humans but only in limited amounts, therefore, a source of EPA and DHA is recommended, either from eating fish or from taking supplements.

The essential oils EPA and DHA have been found to be beneficial to cardiovascular health, brain function and many other processes in the body. They are essential to cell membrane activity and, therefore, affect almost any process in the body.

Saturated fats are also essential to cell function because they constitute a large amount of the bulk of cell membranes and help the omega-3 chains to function properly.

This is where we come to trans-fats (Tip 73). These are modified fats and exist in our food types (especially processed food) for convenience and preservation. They are not good at all. They mimic certain types of fats that the body is used to and perform the wrong functions in their place, contributing to a wide range of problems, particularly inflammation (which can contribute to worse problems, including cardiovascular and Alzheimer's diseases).

The best advice is to stick to natural, unprocessed oils. So what are the best oils to cook with? This is where we should not be using unsaturated oils. The double bonds in the carbon chains, although healthy for us at room temperature, rapidly break down into potentially toxic components when heated. The most healthy oil to cook with is coconut oil (the most heavily saturated oil). A disadvantage is that this leaves a distinct taste in the food that is not always palatable. Butter is probably second best, followed by olive oil due to its relatively high omega-9 content compared with omega-6. For those who want to cook meat in oil, peanut and canola oil can be used, as they have relatively low omega-6 content compared with many other vegetable oils, and add less flavour.

However, the best advice is not to fry food at all (particularly fish due to its high omega-3 content) and bake it in the oven instead – alternatively, fry on a low heat, using butter or coconut oil and added water.

If using cold oils (for example, on salads), virgin olive oil is one of the best; it contains certain polyphenols and other chemicals which are very beneficial to our health.

Tip 64: Vitamin D

Having the right amount of vitamin D is essential to good health. The most natural source of vitamin D is sunlight. But many of us just don't get enough. Whether you can get enough from sunlight or not will highly depend on your lifestyle, but don't take any chances and pop a supplement every day.

Mark Sisson goes into depth on this subject and it is well worth reading. It is possible to take too much, so get tested first and then adjust the dosage depending on your level of acquired sunlight. See http://www.marksdailyapple.com/vitamin-d-sun-exposure-supplementation-and-doses

Tip 65: Nut butters

All low-carb diets allow the consumption of nut butters. Of course, you must choose the varieties that are not full with sugar and other additives, but dipping a lump of celery or a carrot into nut butter can be a nice low-carb snack.

The most common form is peanut butter (note that the peanut is a legume not a nut) but you can get almost every other variety, for example, almond butter or cashew butter. Some are lower in GI than others (see Appendix B).

But you do have to be a bit careful. Nut butters, like nuts, do not tend to fill you up and can make you hungrier. They are also very high in calories. Now we know we say: 'it's not about calories' all the time, but they can have an effect if you get enough of them and nuts/nut butters are very high.

74

So, keep it to one to two tablespoons a day. Note that you can also use nut butters in a whole host of low-carb dessert recipes. For Richard, nuts and nut butters are a problem: he has to stay away from them unless he wants to consume vast amounts. He often has a whole bag of cashews on binge day though – pure bliss...

If you're trying to gain muscle, then a great shake to have when you get up and just before bed is: ½ scoop of whey protein blended with ½ a pint of milk, a spoonful of almond butter and a banana, but this is definitely not recommended for those trying to lose fat!

Tip 66: Muscle gain

There is a lot of misinformation out there about this subject, maybe because there is a lot of uncertainty about the science. We're not going to make any attempt to explain the different types of muscle training (size, strength, endurance) or the physiology of the muscles – we are in no way experts in those subjects, but we do want to expose some rubbish.

There are also a whole host of reasons why someone may want to increase muscle mass, but the most common reason (whether folk admit it or not), is to look good. We're not going to cover that either.

First of all, increasing one's muscle mass is very difficult. By far the best way to 'get ripped' is to lose the fat that covers the muscles. So many folk work out for hours and hours in the gym but seem to make little progress. They feel fitter and their muscles may get a little harder when tensed, but your muscles will simply not show until you shed the fat that covers them. You are much better off concentrating on that, than working on muscle gain.

The exercises for fat loss are not necessarily compatible with muscle mass gain, although resistance work will definitely help you lose fat. Once the fat has gone, you can start a decent resistance training routine and you'll start to see your muscles tone.

To gain any appreciable muscle mass, you have to do two things:

1. You need to train to failure: that is, you need to be doing resistance work which takes you to the point where the muscle fails. For example, a shoulder press where you cannot physically do the final lift. That is the point where the body says 'aha, we need a bit more strength, let's increase our muscle mass'. All the reps you do will make little difference – it is this last failed lift (and holding it at the failure point) where the majority of the work is done. Lots of hormones will then be released to tell the body to grow muscle – all over the body. That's why it's best to concentrate on the big muscle groups, especially the legs.

2. You need to feed the muscle to fuel the growth. And when we say feed, we mean go for it. To get appreciable muscle gain you need to consume vast amounts of food, including carbs.

One thing's for sure, you will not increase muscle mass by going to the gym and doing the same routine every time. You need to increase the resistance force steadily. There is no such thing as just getting ripped by doing loads of reps – you either grow muscle or you don't.

So, lots of training to failure and eating like its Christmas every day (without the sugary stuff). So, guess what happens? You put on fat. It is almost impossible to get appreciable muscle gain without putting on fat. That's why weight lifters are often a little tubby. Bodybuilders go through cycles of gaining muscle, then stripping off fat. They also take copious amounts of drugs, so don't follow their lead.

Here's some numbers for example. In December 2013, Richard did a recommended muscle gain (bulking) programme called Occum's Protocol. You can look it up, but it basically involves lifting like you've got a gun to your head and eating like a mad man. Richard had to be very regimented and spend a fair bit of money on supplements. After 28 days, he gained around 7 kg in total weight, about 3 kg of which was muscle growth. This had a noticeable effect on his body shape and it is remaining now that he has stripped the excess fat off. By the time he got to his natural minimum, he was about 2 kg heavier. So that's a hell of a lot of work just to gain 2 kg of muscle. We'll leave it to you to assess whether it's worth the bother or not.

This year, Richard did the Men's Fitness 16 Week Body Plan. This is a bulking plan designed for tone rather than serious mass gain (it was originally designed to get one of the magazine's editors on the front cover with a full-on six pack). It was seriously hard work – at the end Richard had made very little mass gain, but he was noticeably more toned. He also ignored the advice to use carbs and stayed on the Slow-carb Diet throughout.

That's all we're going to say on this subject. If we could give only one piece of advice it would be to strip fat off before you even consider growing muscle mass.

Tip 67: How to calculate net carbs

Net carbs are the carbohydrates your body will actually absorb from the food you eat.

Here we show you how to calculate net carbs. For non-packaged food items, such as vegetables, fruits and meat, see Appendix A. For packaged foods, see below. Here's a typical food label:

ว sauce. A creamy sauce made wi

Per ½ pot

Calories	Fat	Saturates	Salt	Sugars
142	13.2g	8.2g	0.60g	1.1g

Nutrition waitrose.com/nutrition

Typical values as consumed	per ½ pot	per 100g
Energy	586kJ 142kcal	586kJ 142kcal
Protein	1.9g	1.9g
Carbohydrate	3.3g	3.3g
of which sugars	1.1g	1.1g
Fat	13.2g	13.2g
of which saturates	8.2g	8.2g
Fibre	1.1g	1.1g
Sodium	0.24g	0.24g

Most labels have a column of figures per portion and per 100 g/ml.

We are interested in the portion we will be eating. In this case, it's a creamy sauce, of which we'll enjoy half a pot on a juicy steak!

Calculating net carbs is easy:

In the UK and EU, the figure for carbohydrates **IS** the net carbs. There is nothing to calculate!

In the United States though:

Net carbs   = carbohydrate - fibre

$$= 3.3 \text{ g} - 1.1 \text{ g}$$

Net carbs   = 2.2 g (for half a pot of this sauce)

We took away the fibre (1.1 g) from total carbohydrates (3.3 g) to get the net carbs.

If you choose to count carbs, aim for 35 g net carbs per day in order to start losing weight. You can increase this a little once you see you are losing weight. Everybody's metabolism is different, and some may be able to eat 60 g net carbs a day and still lose weight.

For each item you eat, you would then check the net carbs (tip: meat and eggs are zero net carbs).

Note, when looking at the nutritional information, we are not interested in calories nor are we worried about fat. In fact, if the net carbs are low but fat is high, this is an ideal food for our diet. Fat is our new fuel. That is a key concept of a low-carb diet.

Here's another example:

Per 150ml serving				
Calories	Fat	Saturates	Salt	Sugars
70	0.0g	0.0g	0.00g	16.8g

Nutrition		waitrose.com/nutrition
Typical values as sold	per 150ml serving	per 100ml
Energy	297kJ	198kJ
	70kcal	47kcal
Protein	0.2g	0.1g
Carbohydrate	16.8g	11.2g
of which sugars	16.8g	11.2g
Fat	0.0g	0.0g
of which saturates	0.0g	0.0g
Fibre	0.0g	0.0g
Sodium	0.00g	0.00g

This time it is a carton of apple juice, which is on the AVOID list. We are interested in the 150 millilitre (ml) serving figures.

For the US, Net carbs = carbohydrate – fibre

= 16.8 g – 0 g

Net carbs = 16.8 g (for a glass of juice)

We took away the fibre (0 g) from total carbohydrates (16.8 g) to get the net carbs. In the UK and EU, we simply use the carbohydrate figure on the label.

As the above calculation shows, fruit juice is OUT! If we are aiming for 35 g net carbs per day, this one glass of juice will use up over half our daily allowance.

Tip 68: The Japanese diet

This is not so much a tip as an argument you will need in your back pocket to fend off the unbelievers. We often get asked how the Japanese can stay so trim despite seeming to eat a diet high in carbs (mainly rice and noodles). We have given this much thought and read a little. So, here's our thoughts on the issue.

1. They don't eat large quantities of rice, and don't tend to snack after the evening meal. Rice amounts are usually small compared to, for example, Indian meals. They culturally restrict carbs in the evening, even if sub-consciously. We're not convinced about this argument.
2. They eat three square meals and don't snack so much. It is not the done thing to snack at work or school. Might be a factor?
3. They eat lots of fermented veg. Tim Ferriss is clear in his book about the fat-busting properties of fermented food.
4. They simply eat less than Westerners and there is not so much social pressure to have a curvy (female) or muscular (male) body.
5. They are starting to catch up with us on the fat front, especially their kids.
6. They have a very low consumption of sugar. We think this is significant.
7. They eat low amounts of polyunsaturated fatty acids (PUFA).
8. They drink a lot of green tea. There is some research suggesting that green tea has weight control properties.

So, the combination of less overall carbs (less glycaemic load) than a typical Westerner, less sugar and less PUFA, means that they don't pile on the pounds. Also, there may be a case of always eating protein with carbs (in the past by way of high-protein beans and rice, but more likely meat/fish and rice nowadays).

Clearly, there is more to this game than just cutting out carbs, but that is still the most effective way to get fat off and reach a balance point. At that point, you can experiment to find your carb tolerance, mix things up a bit and see what happens. You won't go far wrong by just going back to how your grandparents used to eat!

This is a seriously interesting subject for us and we would value your thoughts on it. Who knows, one day we may actually have evidence-based nutritional advice from our government that actually makes us healthy (Sweden have). Maybe that's just a little too much to ask...

Tip 69: Yerba Mate tea

Tim Ferriss recommends using Yerba Mate tea to promote bowel movements on binge day (the idea is that all the high-carb stuff you are eating just goes straight through you). But, as with green tea, there are many benefits to Yerba Mate tea.

Yerba mate has been used for centuries by many traditional folk in subtropical South America and is now popular all over the world. It is reported to have many beneficial health effects and is considered a medicine in many cultures. Some of the listed benefits include (and there are many more):

1. Helps weight loss due to its thermogenic properties.
2. Relieves allergies and sinusitis.
3. It's an antioxidant.
4. Strengthens the heart (as it contains theophylline).
5. Boosts the immune system.
6. Aids digestion (this is Tim's point).
7. It is an anti-inflammatory.
8. It lowers blood pressure.
9. It is diuretic.
10. It contains various vitamins and minerals.
11. It is a stimulant – it contains caffeine (this can be good and bad).
12. It can apparently reduce skin wrinkles when the leaves are mashed in a poultice and applied.

It is also reputed to relieve depression and anxiety and aid concentration. There are also horror stories on the internet about Yerba Mate causing cancer and liver disease, but these appear to be in people who literally drink it all day and, even then, the effects are not proven scientifically.

Richard drinks it on binge day and days off work (it takes a little preparation). And of course, you can buy it on Amazon these days.

Justin drinks it occasionally too, but he can't be bothered with all the paraphernalia which goes with it (gourds and straws). He found a nifty little in-cup tea strainer online which works very well. Justin's not a huge caffeine fan and so naturally limits the amount he will drink in a day.

Tip 70: Low-carb and endurance sports

Most people are coming round to the idea of a low-carb diet for weight loss. It is clearly the most effective, healthy and sustainable way to trim down. But many people are not convinced about low-carb for endurance sports (for example, triathlon or long-distance running/cycling.).

The evidence seems to point in the direction of improved performance with a low-carb diet. There is a lot more to it than this, but let's do some simple maths. You can store around 2000 kcals of glycogen. If glycogen is your primary fuel source, once that is used up (if you are not keto-adapted), you will start to take energy from fat and muscle (much less efficiently). But even a lean person has around 40,000 kcals of fat available for energy. If you are keto-adapted, you can tap straight into this source.

Endurance athletes often talk of hitting the 'wall' or 'bonking'. This is where you completely run out of steam and is caused by a lack of glycogen to the brain. It's not very nice and Richard can tell you that from experience. Again, if you are keto-adapted, you will not hit a wall unless you go for days!

There is also an argument that glycogen is somehow a more efficient fuel source, but this is not backed up by evidence. In fact, keto-adapted athletes claim to have more energy, more clarity and more dedication.

It certainly changed Richard's life dramatically. He used to carb-load before races, but no longer needs to.

The only deleterious effect of low-carb that we can find is a slight reduction in top-end 'burst' performance. Sprinters may need some carbs, but endurance athletes do not.

The only words of caution we would give (based on the experience of some friends), is do not keto-adapt during the peak of your training. Adapt out of season or just take a couple of weeks off training whilst you adapt (it only takes a couple of weeks). A great book on the subject is *The Art and Science of Low Carbohydrate Performance* by Stephen Phinney and Jeff Volek.

Tip 71: Fasting

This seems to be a popular subject these days, especially with the apparent short-term success of the 5:2 diet. Fasting is good for you – there are many studies that show large health benefits from intermittent fasting, whether it is just skipping a meal or going without for a whole day.

Humans are perfectly adapted to fasting and we're sure it was pretty normal for our ancestors. We skip the odd meal, but have never tried a whole day – we simply love food too much and find the stress too much! We see no point in starving yourself on a regular basis when there is no need.

Apparently, it does get easier with practice. Also, the fact is that diets should never be seen as quick fixes; they have to be sustainable life changes. And, in our case, starving ourselves twice a week just doesn't cut the biscuit (if you'll pardon the pun). Richard does, however, skip breakfast, and sometimes lunch after a binge day – he finds this very easy as he's packed full of stored glycogen. This helps to bring on ketosis/lipolysis faster (he tested this with keto-sticks and it does work).

As an advanced fat loss tip, you can do some interval training in conjunction with the post-binge day fast, then go for a nice long walk. So, by all means experiment with intermittent fasting, but not at the expense of your quality of life.

Tip 72: Yeast and probiotics

Yeast feeds on sugar. With a diet rich in sugar and refined carbohydrates, many people unknowingly suffer from an overgrowth of yeast in their intestines.

If you suffer from constant headaches, feeling foggy, lethargy, gas or bloating you may be suffering from a yeast imbalance. Cutting down on carbs will certainly help with this, but you may need a helping hand in the form of probiotics.

Probiotics are beneficial bacteria which are able to deal with a yeast (*Candida albicans*) overgrowth. Find a good-quality probiotic, which contains acidophilus, bulgaricus and bifidobacterium. Take these regularly until symptoms subsist. Be aware also that all antibiotics have an effect on your bowel flora. A strong course of antibiotics will leave you wide open to a yeast overgrowth, so be sure to take probiotics during and after treatment.

Whilst natural yoghurts contain an amount of beneficial bacteria, it is better to take a good-quality capsule if you suspect a yeast overgrowth. Bio-Kult is one such supplement which has very good reviews online. Justin believes he has eliminated his son's IBS through the use of probiotics.

Tip 73: Trans-fats

These are a nasty kind of fat that has the double whammy effect of lowering your good cholesterol levels (HDL) and raising your bad ones (LDL). Trans-fats (or trans-fatty acid) are made by adding hydrogen to vegetable oil through a process called hydrogenation, which makes the oil less likely to spoil. Using trans-fats in the manufacturing of foods helps foods stay fresh longer, have a longer shelf-life and have a less greasy feel. We aren't sure exactly why, but the addition of hydrogen to oil increases your LDL more than other types of fats do.

How do you know whether food contains trans-fats? Trans-fats are (or have been – their use is decreasing) been found in many processed foods for example, biscuits and cakes, chips/fries, crisps and ready meals. On food labels, look for the words 'partially hydrogenated' vegetable oil. That's another term for trans-fats. It sounds counterintuitive, but 'fully' or 'completely' hydrogenated oil doesn't contain trans-fats. Unlike partially hydrogenated oil, the process used to make fully or completely hydrogenated oil doesn't result in trans-fatty acids. However, if the label says just 'hydrogenated' vegetable oil, it could mean the oil contains some trans-fats. Although small amounts of trans-fat occur naturally in some meat and dairy products, it's the trans-fats in processed foods that are most harmful. Note that you should of course be avoiding all forms of vegetable or seed oil anyway (see Tip 11).

Tip 74: Omega-3 part 2

Algae/phytoplankton oil supplements are a purer source of these omega-3 oils (this is how most of it gets into the fish in the first place), suitable for vegetarians and good for lots of other reasons because of the wide range of phytonutrients in them, but they're not a cheap option.

As a good source of EPA and DHA, the best type of fish is salmon. Wild Atlantic or Pacific salmon is far better than farmed salmon for many reasons, including the fact that the artificial diet that the farmed fish are fed on decreases the omega-3/omega-6 ratio. Always look for sustainably sourced labels on fish products if you care about the environment.

Herrings and mackerel have almost as much omega-3 as salmon. Tinned tuna, however, contains virtually none of these oils; the way it is cooked removes them before being canned. Tinned sardines, herring, mackerel or wild salmon are okay.

Reports about the dangers of omega-3 oils were based on flawed (and possibly biased) research. The reason for keeping these supplements in the fridge and away from light is that heavily conjugated (unsaturated) oils oxidise easily and will quickly go rancid. Gelatin capsules are not so much of an issue as there is much less exposure to oxygen but should still be kept away from sunlight.

Another note of caution: the best way to cook fish is to bake it in the oven and without overcooking. Pan frying, although a tasty way of cooking fish, can destroy much of the EPA and DHA content because of the high temperatures involved.

Tip 75: A new plateau buster

We gave some ideas about weight loss plateaux in Tip 39. It's something almost everyone will face. There are a number of methods to beat them (including just patience), but this is one you may like: a three-day binge. Yes, you heard it; three days of eating anything you want is enough to shock your body out of a plateau. Obviously, don't try this unless you have seen no weight loss for a few weeks or if you are near your natural minimum. Have fun!

Tip 76: Salt

As your body adjusts to its new low-carb regime, your liver will start to operate differently and you will begin to shed your electrolytes at a higher rate (you should be peeing more also as you are drinking more water, or should be). Tim Ferriss suggests taking extra doses of potassium, magnesium and sodium, but a good general purpose vitamin and mineral supplement should do most of the trick.

See Tip 54 for more advice on salt.

Tip 77: Free radicals – the silent killers

Free radicals are highly reactive atoms with an odd number of electrons. These are formed in the body as a result of normal metabolic processes. They can also be ingested in the form of cigarette smoke, pollution or burnt food.

They present a real danger to our cell membranes and components such as DNA. Being highly reactive, they can start a chain reaction which can damage or kill a cell. Also, if DNA is damaged then cancer can result.

The body has a mechanism to deal with free radicals, and these are called antioxidants. You have probably seen adverts stating that a certain food is high in antioxidants.

Antioxidants really are our friends. Foods which are rich in them will do you good. Blueberries, strawberries, raspberries and blackberries have high levels, as do kale and spinach. Vitamin C and E are powerful antioxidants.

Berries and cream, perhaps with a sprinkling of flax seed, is a delicious dessert – and you can eat it often, knowing you are helping your health in every way.

Tip 78: What is too much protein?

There have been claims that high-protein diets are as bad for you as smoking. The first thing to bear in mind for us low-carbers is that a low-carb diet should NOT be a high protein diet. You should be eating no more protein than a 'normal' diet.

If you want to add muscle mass or are training for something that involves constantly ripping muscle fibres, then you need to increase protein that, but only for short periods.

It is worth noting that too much protein can actually be converted into fat by a process known as nucleogenesis, so it is best to keep it at a balanced level. Most low-carb diets recommend 0.8 – 2 g of protein per kilogram of bodyweight, but this will vary with age, sex and activity level, so do some reading around the subject.

But the crucial message here is: low-carb dieting is not high-protein dieting so don't think you can just stuff down huge steaks each meal.

Tip 79: A fat-burning tip

Exercise is not a very effective way of burning fat. Diet is by far the most effective way to lose the kilos.

However, to maximise fat loss through exercise, you should work out before breakfast. That way, all glycogen stores will have been used up in the night, and you'll get straight down to fat burning.

We're not suggesting long CV sessions before breakfast (that will make you tired in the day), but a short high-intensity session or just a thirty minute power walk will burn a little extra fat. If you fancy taking the dog for a stroll or hitting the park in the morning for some sprints before breakfast, go for it; it's a great way to start the day.

Tip 80: Garlic

Garlic is a true superfood and you should try to eat it as often as possible. If the odour is an issue, odourless capsules can be taken.

Garlic contains allicin, a powerful antioxidant which helps limit the damage from free radicals. It also boosts the immune system, lowers blood pressure and reduces cholesterol. It is an excellent source of vitamin B6, manganese, selenium and vitamin C. Several studies suggest that garlic reduces the likelihood of blood platelets sticking to artery walls, thus reducing the risk of a heart attack.

If you have been avoiding garlic, now is the time to change!

Tip 81: Hormones

It is possible to follow a low-carb lifestyle and not understand the science behind it. However, certainly in Richard's case (he is a scientist), he finds it very important to know what's going on. We want some convincing and some good arguments to bring up in discussions with 'unbelievers'.

Hormones are an important part of the story. Hormones are defined in the *Oxford English Dictionary* as 'regulatory substances produced in an organism and transported in tissue fluids such as blood to stimulate specific cells or tissues into action'. We can't better that or put it more simply. Now we're going to tell you about the three most important hormones involved in our eating. We'll start with the one we've all heard of: insulin.

Tip 82: Insulin

Oxford English Dictionary definition: 'a hormone produced in the pancreas by the islets of Langerhans, which regulates the amount of glucose in the blood'. When we eat carbs, they are broken down in the body into glucose, which enters the bloodstream. The glucose or 'blood sugar' can be used for immediate energy requirements or , thanks to insulin, can be shipped to the liver, muscle and fat cells to be stored for later use as glycogen.

In a healthy person, insulin is released in proportions that are appropriate to the level of blood sugar. Basically, if the level of blood sugar is higher than is required for energy, it will get stored as fat. That's it. Control blood sugar spikes, and you'll control fat production – that's the basis of all low-carb diets.

So why can't someone just tell us the level of carbs to eat and we'll all be okay? The answer is: we're all different. Your 'carb tolerance' will depend on fitness level, general health, metabolism, age, sex and nutritional history. We have to self-experiment, but in general, if you stick to the foods listed in your chosen low-carb eating regime, you should be okay. You can then try raising the carb amount and see what happens.

As well as blood sugar spikes, insulin resistance is also an issue. When our bodies have to permanently produce copious amounts of insulin to clear the excess glucose, the insulin receptors can become less efficient. As a result, more and more insulin is secreted to get the job done and it will now take even more insulin to communicate that the glucose needs to be cleared. Also, the excess glucose hangs about in the blood. This is what we call high blood sugar – a determining factor in the prognosis of diabetes.

Overconsumption of carbs can cause blood sugar spikes, insulin resistance and high blood sugar – all potentially leading to obesity, diabetes, cancer, and a whole host of other 'modern' diseases.

We need to get control of the insulin in our lives or reap the consequences.

Tip 83: Leptin

Oxford English Dictionary definition: 'a protein produced by fatty tissue which is believed to regulate fat storage in the body'. Leptin is the major hormone involved in appetite regulation and has the important job of stopping you starving to death.

When food is scarce, leptin levels increase, signalling to the body to down-regulate our metabolism to protect us from starvation (i.e. to hold on to fat stores). This was fine when we lived in caves. But these days, food is everywhere, unless you go on a typical low-calorie diet (i.e. starve yourself). Restrict calories = leptin levels drop = hold on to fat, i.e. bad news.

Another way leptin levels can drop is through weight loss itself. When we lose fat, we naturally lose the quantity of leptin (which is secreted by fat cells) we once had working in our favour. That's why it gets more and more difficult to lose fat with time, especially the 'last few pounds'.

Also, when leptin drops, we feel hungry. Therefore, any diet that decreases leptin is going right against the grain, which is why the failure rate is so high.

The trick is to manipulate leptin to maintain a healthy level which will allow you to keep your metabolism burning high and allow fat stores to be burned. And guess what, that's a low-carb diet.

Note that a good binge day will result in increased leptin. That's one of the reasons you should really go for it and eat until you are stuffed on binge day.

Tip 84: Ghrelin

We've come to the last of our important hormones. *Oxford English Dictionary* definition: 'a gastrointestinal hormone produced by epithelial cells lining the fundus of the stomach; appears to be a stimulant for appetite and feeding, but is also a strong stimulant of growth hormone secretion from the anterior pituitary'. This is another appetite regulation hormone, which also has the job of keeping us from starvation.

Ghrelin is a bit like the inverse of insulin. When insulin levels are high, ghrelin levels will be low. But when insulin levels are low, ghrelin comes in to play – it tells our brain that our stomach is empty and we need food fast. Ideally, a good diet would maintain levels of insulin (and hence blood sugar), leptin and ghrelin. No prizes for guessing the best way of eating to do that.

Tip 85: Protein shakes and fasting

Intermittent fasting is a way of speeding up your weight loss programme. It comes in a range of types (for example, 24 hours, 4-hour window, Warrior diet, 5:2) and is very healthy. People report better focus and productivity during a fast, and the physical benefits have been well documented. But a question that comes up is whether protein shakes can be taken whilst fasting. The simple answer is no, definitely not. If you are drinking protein during a fast, you are not fasting, you are following a short high-protein diet, which can be dangerous.

Tip 86: Eating out

If you enjoy meat, poultry or seafood, you really shouldn't have any problem when eating out. Delicious steaks, fish and even luxury foods such as lobster and crab are available to you. Just avoid the carbs lying around, such as bread. Instead of bread while you peruse the menu, perhaps ask for a bowl of olives instead.

For meals which come with potatoes or fries, most chefs will happily oblige a request to replace them with extra vegetables.

At Indian restaurants, just leave out the rice and breads. You'll be surprised how much you enjoy curries without the rice, along with a side dish or two of vegetables. Carb-rich foods, such as rice, have a tendency to make you overeat. When you leave them out, you will feel pleasantly full without feeling bloated – the usual unpleasant feeling after an Indian meal.

If you have no option but to grab something at a fast-food restaurant, grab a double burger with cheese and bacon and discard the roll. Get that with a salad but avoid the dressing as it's bound to be full of sugar.

Tip 87: Low-carb bread

There are now several brands of low-carb bread on the market, which are very good. The two examples we use are Hi-Lo from Sainsbury's and Liv-Life from Waitrose. You can also get them from Amazon (although it's a little expensive).

There are others labelled 'lower carb' eg Hovis which are still pretty high carb and you need to be careful with them, or avoid them.

Tip 88: Cauliflower rice

For those of you that miss rice, especially with a curry, there is a nice alternative. Take a cauliflower and bash it up in a blender. Then pop it in a sealed container, add some salt, and microwave on full for eight minutes.

To be honest, we have been low carb for so long now that we don't really look for alternatives for anything. We're happy with protein and veg, but occasionally a rice alternative is nice.

Note that it doesn't taste too much like cauliflower for some reason – certainly not in an overpowering way. Happy cooking.

Tip 89: Food combining – protein and fat

Combining different foods in certain ways can have either a positive or negative effect on blood sugar levels (and hence, insulin production and, in turn, fat storage). The first combination we shall consider is the best one: protein and fat. Neither protein nor fat has much effect on blood sugar levels. Eating protein with fat (for example, a juicy steak slavering in garlic herb butter) will give you the amino acids to maintain and build muscle, and fill you up (keep your ghrelin levels low). Of course, remember not to eat too much protein as this can lead to blood sugar spikes. So, protein with fat is a good combination.

Tip 90: Food combining – protein and carbs

We know that eating carbs is not good if you are trying to lose weight and an excess (the normal amount for most people) can lead to a whole host of diseases. And we know that protein doesn't have a negative effect on blood sugar (unless over-consumed). But, if you eat protein with carbs, your insulin level will not increase as much as if you just ate the carbs. Once we are keto-adapted, we can get away with eating some carbs in our diet, if we eat them with some protein. However, whilst trying to drop weight, just cut them out (until binge day of course) and wait until you get to your natural minimum. Once there, you can experiment and see what you can get away with.

Tip 91: Food combining – carbs and fat

You should remember that carbs send the blood sugar through the roof and that fat has virtually no effect on it. But, if we eat carbs with fat, you do not get the same carb-limiting effect that you get with protein. In fact, you see an even bigger spike in insulin than you would with the carbs alone. This is pretty much the only scenario where dietary fat is shuttled directly to your fat cells (stored). The carbs cause the doors to your fat cells to open, and the fat gets a free ride in. So, for example, if you ate pancakes with butter, pretty much the entire energy content of the food would be stored as fat (assuming you have no immediate requirement for that energy). We think this, combined with carb-only eating, is the key issue with obesity around the world. Take home message: never eat refined carbs alone or refined carbs with fat. Of course, many of us do this on binge day – that's why you should follow the steps suggested by Tim Ferriss to minimise the effects (see Tip 42).

Tip 92: Stress and weight loss

It has been said that stress was a great way of losing weight, but many folk state that it has the opposite effect. The link is normally made with the stress hormone, cortisol. Cortisol does have the potential to affect your rate of weight loss. But it's not as simple as saying that when cortisol goes up, your rate of weight loss goes down. Nor is it the case that suppressing cortisol will help you lose weight — as the people trying to sell you cortisol-blocking supplements would have you believe.

Cortisol has firmly established itself as one of the 'villains' in the hormonal world of goodies and baddies. But actually, it isn't. In the right amount and at the right time, cortisol has several benefits for anyone wanting more muscle and less fat. Firstly, cortisol has anti-inflammatory properties. It doesn't cause inflammation, but rises in response to inflammation. This gives it an important role to play in repairing muscle damage after exercise.

But if cortisol levels are high for long periods of time, for example during periods of high stress, there can be problems.

Note that a high-exercise, restricted-diet regime will cause significant stress to the body. However, cortisol has the ability to make us retain more water, so often the weight gain you see is not due to fat storage.

The only way to dissipate cortisol is to rest and eat good food, although many people are under the impression that you should exercise heavily. But this will set up a vicious circle. You should address the stress-causing factors in your life, not chase around trying to drive them away. A prolonged elevation in cortisol isn't great news for your muscles either.

Also, cortisol inhibits protein synthesis and promotes protein breakdown, as well as countering the effects of other anabolic hormones, testosterone in particular. Cortisol makes your brain less sensitive to the effects of leptin, blunting its satiating signal. This can leave you feeling a lot hungrier than normal.

Cortisol also tends to stimulate your appetite, particularly for foods that are high in starch, sugar or fat (if you combine with the carbs).

Not everyone will experience all these effects and some people actually lose their appetite due to stress. We don't want to create the impression that a rise in cortisol levels somehow makes weight gain inevitable, because that certainly isn't always the case.

Combining massive amounts of exercise with an extremely restrictive diet in a frantic attempt to lose as much fat as you can in as little time as possible is not a great idea. But cutting out exercise completely because you've read a bunch of 'scare stories' about what it's going to do to you is also a mistake.

The truth can be found somewhere in the middle. The best advice is not to get over-stressed in the first place and learn other non-exercise/diet methods for dealing with it. Learn about the subject, look at your life and try things like yoga, meditation, a good hobby, a decent holiday, or simply facing your problems and dealing with them.

Tip 93: Chronic cardio

Cardio is an indispensable part of any exercise regime. However, many people go over the top in a vain attempt to use masses of cardio to lose weight. It can also be very addictive due to the feelings of wellbeing post exercise (everyone says this is down to endorphins but this is not a proven fact). We know people who have literally become clinically depressed on being told to stop, for example, running.

If you are training for a specific endurance event, then running/cycling/rowing/etc. for long distances or times (chronic) cardio is a must. But if you are not in training for something, it is not necessarily good for you. Yes, if you really push it, you will lose mass – but you will lose fat and muscle at the same time.

Plus, the body soon gets used to this way of exercising. It will alter your metabolism accordingly and you'll start losing less mass. If you want to lose mass, you are much better off concentrating on what you eat.

Chronic cardio is very stressful on your muscles, ligaments and bones and often leads to niggling or crippling injuries (Richard had to have a knee operation after pounding the streets for years). Also, because it is stressful, it will cause the release of hormones (mainly cortisol) which can get in the way of mass loss (see Tip 82).

If you just want to be fit and healthy, then one interval session per week and two to five hours of easy cardio is all you need. The easy stuff can just be walking or cycling to work if you wish.

Tip 94: Breakfast 2

We covered breakfast in Tip 8, but here's some more information about why, in general, you should not skip breakfast.

When you skip breakfast, among the many other negative things that happen is that insulin release is greater at the next meal than it would otherwise have been. Blood sugar is destabilised and you're more likely to be subject to cravings. In all likelihood, you're running on empty and masking it with coffee/tea.

If you're one of those people who have no appetite in the morning, it's probably because you've conditioned yourself to this unnatural way of eating. A good place to start with the rehabilitation of your appetite is with a protein shake. Even people who are not hungry in the morning can handle a shake, especially if it's delicious and made with good extras like berries or a tablespoon of nut butter.

Eventually, you should transition to a whole-food breakfast (at least for most days), and make sure it contains protein and some good fats. If you need some additional motivation: several studies have found a correlation between being overweight and skipping breakfast. The only time we skip breakfast is the day after a binge day – this is perfectly acceptable as you are brimming with glycogen. It's a great time to go do some exercise too.

Tip 95: Potassium

This is an essential chemical for the body. If you are feeling tired too often, getting cramps, constipation, dry skin or irritability, this could be down to a lack of potassium. Serious deficiency can be highly dangerous.

Low-carb eating tends to cause the liver to kick out more electrolyte salts (the reason you need to increase your salt intake when you go low-carb). Potassium has multiple roles in the body. To name but a few: regulating fluids, regulating blood pressure, waste removal, controlling the dynamics of electrical impulses around the body and, importantly for us, ketogenesis.

If you fear you are not getting enough potassium, then there are some good whole-food sources. Some examples include: yogurt (not allowed on the Slow-carb Diet of course), spinach, avocado, broccoli, mushrooms, lentils, salmon and all meat (especially pork). Note that if you are getting your potassium from meat, make sure you eat the juices you cook the meat in – the potassium has a habit of leaching out. Actually, a good general tip is to always eat the lovely fat and other juices that come off meat. Also check out Lo-Salt which is a table salt that includes potassium.

Bananas are also a great source of potassium but are a very high-carb fruit, and should definitely be avoided if you are trying to lose body fat. And, after all that, if you can't be bothered cooking, just take a supplement.

Tip 96: Magnesium

Magnesium is another essential chemical for health. Magnesium helps regulate over 300 reactions in the body, including your energy balance and metabolism.

Deficiency will result in many of the symptoms discussed for potassium. Good sources include avocado, all green veg, salmon, mackerel, flax seed, almonds, sunflower seeds and all meats. Again, you can supplement if you wish or even use Epsom salts in the bath.

Richard used to suffer from bad night cramps and finally cured them by, first, taking high doses of magnesium and then settling on whole-food sources.

Tip 97: Glycogen store

Even if you are keto-adapted (following a low-carb diet), you will still have a store of sugar (glycogen) which is used as a sort of immediate energy source, and is integral to muscle growth. This will come from the complex carbs you are eating (veg, legumes) and from protein synthesis. So, if you really want to be efficient at burning fat, do some high-intensity activity (for example, some serious lifting or interval training), then go for a nice long walk. You will deplete your store and then burn purely fat. It's also a good idea to burn off your store before and after a binge day.

This is one of the reasons why interval training is so effective: it can leave you burning off pure fat for days. This is also why chronic cardio is so ineffective: you are simply burning off your store.

Tip 98: Ketoacidosis and ketosis

Ketoacidosis (or diabetic ketoacidosis) is a potentially life-threatening complication in patients with diabetes. It happens predominantly in those with type 1 diabetes, but it can occur in those with type 2 diabetes under certain circumstances.

Ketoacidosis results from a shortage of insulin; in response the body switches to burning fatty acids and producing acidic ketone bodies that cause most of the symptoms and complications. But it is not the same as ketosis, and don't let anyone tell you it is.

Ketosis is the condition that can be reached when restricting dietary carbohydrates, where the body switches over from predominantly burning glycogen (sugars) for fuel and instead burning fat. This switch means the liver produces ketones for bodily fuel (including for the brain).

But the amount of ketones produced is nowhere near as many as in ketoacidosis. Keto-adaptation is the process of making the switch and usually takes about two weeks of carb restriction. In our (and many much more qualified folk's) opinion, it is a healthier state than being glycogen fuelled and is our natural state.

Many can feel when they are in a ketogenic state. It's hard to explain – they just know. We most definitely have more energy, concentration, focus and feelings of wellbeing.

Tip 99: Why is HIIT so effective?

There is no doubt that high-intensity interval training is a very effective way to reach peak fitness levels and burn fat. There are many ways to do HIIT. But for now, the easiest way is to get yourself up to 85-100% effort for a few seconds (say 20-30 s to start), then rest (walk, jog, slow cycle) until you get your breath back (say 30–60 s), and repeat a few times. Spinning is another good method.

There are literally hundreds of methods, so do some internet research and talk to your trainer. But, why is it so effective?

1. More energy expenditure. Intervals are not easy – you will always be exerting more effort than chronic cardio.
2. Uses your glycogen store for energy (so you can get straight to fat burning afterwards, sometimes for days).
3. Increases production of lactic acid – this in turn increases growth hormone production, which promotes stored fat usage.
4. Allows for a huge range of workout options – stops you getting bored.
5. Ups metabolic rate for up to two days – the so called 'afterburn' effect.

And we're sure there are others – please let us know if you know any.

You do have to be a little careful not to do too much though. Take at least one rest day in between HIIT sessions. Also, HIIT can be quite stressful and we have discussed the issues with this. If you just want to be fit, one session a week will do. The good news is that 20 minutes HIIT can be more effective than one hour pounding the pavement destroying your limbs.

Tip 100: Detox diets

The idea that the body needs some form of detoxification diet is not correct. It is pure marketing so don't be taken in. The very idea that the body somehow needs help to get rid of toxins has absolutely no basis in biology.

Your organs and immune system handle detox duties, no matter what you eat. Plus, a lot of the so-called healthy detox diets are more harmful than beneficial. Most people don't feel good on low-calorie, nutrient-poor diets. Potential side effects include low energy, low blood sugar, muscle aches, fatigue, feeling dizzy or lightheaded and nausea.

Without doubt, the best thing you can do for your body is to reduce the amount of refined carbohydrates you eat. This will improve your fat loss, insulin tolerance and immune response, plus reduce your chances of diabetes, heart disease, cancer, Alzheimer's, depression – the list goes on and on. Short-term diets do not work. Change your life instead.

Appendix A: Carbohydrate content of common foods

In this appendix we give you a rough idea of the carbohydrate content of many common foods. During your weight loss, we recommend that you do not exceed 35 net carbs per day. Both low- and high-carb foods are listed here. Look at the net carbs column and you will easily spot the foods to include and exclude in order to stay 'low-carb'.

MEAT AND MEAT SUBSTITUTES

Cooked meat is allowed and you can eat it until you are full. Avoid anything in breadcrumbs or other coatings. Beware of pies – toppings and pastry will be full of carbs.

Name	Portion size	Net carbs per portion	Net carbs per 100 g
Bacon	any amount	0	0
Beef (all cuts)	any amount	0	0
Beef minced	any amount	0	0
Chicken	any amount	0	0
Chilli con carne	1 bowl, no rice	22	9
Cornish pasty*	1 pasty	40	25
Duck	any amount	0	0
Kidney	1 kidney	1	1
Lamb (all types)	any amount	0	0
Liver	1 liver	1	1
Meat pie*	1 piece	18	17
Pepperoni	any amount	0	0
Pheasant	any amount	0	0
Pork chop	any amount	0	0
Pork fillet	any amount	0	0

Name	Portion size	Net carbs per portion	Net carbs per 100 g
Pork in frankfurter	1 frankfurter (no roll)	1.4	2
Pork minced	any amount	0	0
Pork pie	1 small	16	25
Pork spare ribs	any amount	0	0
Quorn mince**	1 cup	3	4.5
Quorn sausages**	per sausage	2.7	4.5
Salami	1 slice	0.3	2
Shepherd's pie***	1 bowl	31	14
Steak	any amount	0	0
Tofu (meat alternative)	100 g block	1.6	1.6
Turkey breast	any amount	0	0
Veal	any amount	0	0

*Carbs in the pastry – avoid

**Always check the carbs on package – some may have carbs added elsewhere

***Carbs in the potato - avoid

FISH AND SEAFOOD

Avoid all breaded or battered fish as this adds carbs.

Name	Portion size	Net carbs per portion	Net carbs per 100 g
Crab (cooked)	1 crab	0	0
Fish (any type, plain, cooked)	1 fillet	0	0
Fish (battered)	1 small fillet	21	15
Lobster (plain, cooked)	1 portion	0	0
Prawns	5 medium	0.5	1
Salmon fillet	1 fillet	0	0
Scallops	1 scallop	1	3
Shrimps	10	0.5	1
Trout	1 fillet	0	0
Tuna (fresh or tinned)	any amount	0	0

DAIRY, CHEESE and EGGS

Avoid low-fat varieties – they contain more carbohydrates. Although not dairy, soya milk and almond milk are listed here because they are good alternatives.

Name	Portion size	Net carbs per portion	Net carbs per 100 g
Almond milk (unsweetened)	200 ml glass	0	0
Butter	big chunk	0	0.1
Camembert cheese	3 x 1 inch cubes	0.3	0.5
Cheddar cheese	3 x 1 inch cubes	0.6	1.3
Cottage cheese	4 tablespoons	1	3
Cream (heavy /whipping)	2 tablespoons	1	2.7
Cream (light)	2 tablespoons	1	3.6
Cream (sour)	2 tablespoons	1.5	4
Cream cheese	2 tablespoons	0.6	2.5
Egg (boiled)	1 large	0.6	1.1
Egg (fried)	1 egg	0.4	0.8
Egg (omelette)	3 eggs	1.2	0.6
Egg (poached)	1 egg	0.7	0.7
Egg (scrambled)	4 tablespoons	0.8	1.6
Feta cheese	3 x 1 inch cubes	2	4.1
Goat's cheese	3 x 1 inch cubes	1.2	1.8

Name	Portion size	Net carbs per portion	Net carbs per 100 g
Mascarpone cheese	2 tablespoons	1	1.8
Milk (lactose-free)	200 ml glass	5.6	2.8
Milk (skimmed)	200 ml glass	12	6
Milk (whole)	200 ml glass	10	5
Mozzarella cheese	2 tablespoons	0.6	2.2
Parmesan cheese	2 tablespoons	0.4	4

Name	Portion size	Net carbs per portion	Net carbs per 100 g
Ricotta cheese	3 x 1 inch cubes	1	3
Soya milk (unsweetened)	200 ml glass	0.4	0.2
Swiss cheese	3 x 1 inch cubes	1.2	2
Yogurt, fruit	1 small pot	24	19
Yogurt, Greek, natural	1/2 pot	4	4

VEGETABLES

Potatoes are the number one thing to avoid here.
Check the carbs on the others and you'll soon learn which
are best.

Name	Portion size	Net carbs per portion	Net carbs per 100 g
Artichoke	1 medium	7.5	6
Asparagus spears	five spears	1.5	2
Aubergine	1 medium	2	2.5
Avocado	half a fruit	2	2
Baked potato	1 baked potato	54	17
Beetroot	1 medium	5.5	7
Broccoli	3 florets	4	4
Brussel sprouts	6 sprouts	5	5
Butternut squash	4 tablespoons	10	10
Cabbage	4 large spoonfuls	2	2
Carrot	1 medium	5	6.5
Cauliflower	1 quarter of a head	2	1.8

Name	Portion size	Net carbs per portion	Net carbs per 100 g
Celery	1 medium stalk	0.5	1.5
Chilli pepper (small red)	1 birds eye size	0.1	6
Courgette (Zucchini)	1 small	2.5	2
Cucumber	half of cucumber	2	3.6
Fennel	1 cooked bulb	5	2.5
Garlic	1 clove	1	31
Gherkins	3 pickles	7	21
Green beans	12 beans	2.5	4
Kale (cooked)	1 serving	4	4
Leek	1 medium leek	10.5	12
Lettuce (Cos)	quarter of whole lettuce	1.5	1
Lettuce (round)	quarter of whole lettuce	1.5	1.6
Marrow	100 grams	1.5	1.5
Mushrooms (button)	10 mushrooms	2	3.3
Mushrooms (large)	1 mushroom	0.6	2.3
Mushrooms (medium)	6 mushrooms	2.4	3.3
Okra	8 pods	4	4
Olives	10 olives	2	2.8
Onion	1 medium	7	7
Parsnip	1 large	21	12.5
Peas	4 tablespoons	4	9
Peas (sugar snap)	10 pea pods	1.7	5
Pepper (green)	ten strips	0.5	2.6
Pepper (red)	ten strips	1	4.5
Potato	1 medium	28	14
Potato (mashed)	3 tablespoons	12	12

Name	Portion size	Net carbs per portion	Net carbs per 100 g
Potato (roast)	1 potato	24	18
Potato chips in UK/French fries	1 serving	48	41
Pumpkin	5 tablespoons	6	5.5
Quorn mince	1 cup	3	4.5
Quorn sausages	per sausage	2.7	4.5
Radish	5 medium	0.5	2
Samphire	100 g serving	1.6	1.6
Shallot (echalion)	1 small shallot	4.6	13.8
Spinach (cooked)	4 tablespoons	2	2
Spinach (raw)	big handful	1	1.1
Spring greens	any amount	0	0
Spring onions	1 medium	0.6	4
Swede	quarter whole swede	5	5.6
Sweetcorn	1 medium ear	17	17
Sweet potato	1 small	10	18
Tomato fresh	1 medium whole (2'–3')	3.3	1.7
Tomatoes (tinned)	1 can	6	3
Turnip	1 small turnip	2.8	4.2

FRUIT

You can see that some berries are allowed.
Avoid dried fruits like the plague – they are full of carbs.

Name	Portion size	Net carbs per portion	Net carbs per 100 g
Apple	1 medium	20	12

Name	Portion size	Net carbs per portion	Net carbs per 100 g
Apricot, fresh	1 fruit	3.2	9
Apricot, dried	5 dried fruits	20	55
Avocado	half a fruit	2	2
Banana	1 fruit	24	21
Blackberries	15 fruits	3	5
Blueberries	15 berries	3	11.6
Cantaloupe melon	1 wedge (1/8 fruit)	5	7
Cherries	10 fruits	10	10
Coconut (dried)	30 g	2	8
Coconut (fresh flesh)	2-inch-square piece	3	6
Coconut milk (unsweetened)	4 tablespoons	2	4
Cranberries (dried)	4 tablespoons	31	76
Cranberries, raw	4 tablespoons	4	8
Fig, fresh	1 medium	8.5	16
Grapes	20 grapes	8	16
Honeydew melon	1 wedge (1/8 fruit)	10	8
Kiwi fruit	1 fruit	8	12
Mango	1/2 fruit	22	13
Nectarine	1 medium	12	8.5
Orange	1 medium	12	12
Papaya	1 small fruit	15	9
Pear	1 medium	21	12
Pineapple	1 thick slice	9	11
Plum	1 fruit	7	10
Raspberries	10 large raspberries	3	6
Rhubarb	unsweetened stalk	1.3	2.5
Strawberries	5 medium	3	6
Tangerine	1 medium	11	11

Name	Portion size	Net carbs per portion	Net carbs per 100 g
Watermelon	1 wedge (1/16 fruit)	21	8

BREAD, CEREALS and GRAIN

All breakfast cereals are out, as are breads and rolls. Have bacon and eggs for breakfast instead (see Tip 8).

Name	Portion size	Net carbs per portion	Net carbs per 100 g
Bagel	1 bagel	48	49
Biscuits	2 medium	14	68
Bread (Hi-Lo brand, low-carb)	1 slice	1.6	5.4
Bread (multigrain)	1 slice	13	43
Bread (rye)	1 slice	12	48
Bread (white)	1 slice	15	49
Bulgar wheat	25 g	12	60
Cookies	2 medium	14	68
Corn flour	1 tablespoon	6	70
Cornflakes	1 bowl	28	80
Couscous	30 g	17	45
Croissant	1 croissant	30	46
Doughnut	1 medium	22	50
Flax Seed	1 tablespoon	0.1	2
Flour (almond)	1 tablespoon	0.5	8
Flour (white)	1 tablespoon	6	74
Flour (whole wheat)	1 tablespoon	6	73
French bread	1 slice	18	56
Garlic bread	1 slice	25	42
Pearl barley	25 g	19	80
Pita bread	1 medium	25	56
Pitta bread	1 large	32	54
Porridge oats	1 bowl	20	50
Rice (brown)	small bowl	23	23
Rice (white)	small bowl	28	28
Rice (wild)	small bowl	21	21

Name	Portion size	Net carbs per portion	Net carbs per 100 g
Rice Krispies	1 bowl	29	87
Sandwich	1	26	31
Tortilla	1 tortilla	25	50
Weetabix	2 biscuits	22	59

NUTS

Name	Portion size	Net carbs per portion	Net carbs per 100 g
Almonds	20 nuts	2	5
Brazil	10 nuts	3	4
Cashew	10 nuts	5	26
Honey roast cashews	large handful	12	24
Macadamia	10 nuts	3	5
Peanuts	1 large handful	3	8
Peanuts (dry roasted)	1 large handful	4	14
Pecan	10 halves	1.5	14
Pine	1 tablespoon	0.9	9.5
Pistachio	20 nuts	2	18
Walnuts	10 halves	2	7

PASTA

Name	Portion size	Net carbs per portion	Net carbs per 100 g
Macaroni	1 serving	33	24
Noodles (egg)	1 serving	40	25
Pasta (cooked)	1 serving	30	25
Spaghetti	1 serving	43	31

BEANS

Name	Portion size	Net carbs per portion	Net carbs per 100 g
Baked beans (Heinz)	half normal can	19	9
Black beans	3 tablespoons	18	46
Broad beans	3 tablespoons	4.5	10
Cannellini beans (tinned)	3 tablespoons	2	6
Haricot beans	3 tablespoons	7.2	16
Hummus	3 tablespoons	3.6	8
Lentils	3 tablespoons	4.5	12
Pinto beans	3 tablespoons	18	47
Red kidney beans (tinned)	3 tablespoons	9	21

SOUPS

Check the labels for net carbs as different brands can vary. But if eating out, this guide will help. You'll see that broths are the lowest – they are a good source of salt too.

Name	Portion size	Net carbs per portion	net carbs per 100 g
Beef broth / bouillon	1 mug	0.5	1
Chicken broth / bouillon	1 mug	0.5	1
Chicken noodle soup	1 mug	7.5	3
Chicken soup	1 mug	16	6
Clam chowder	1 mug	17	7
Crab bisque	1 mug	9	4
Cream of asparagus soup	1 mug	13	5

Name	Portion size	Net carbs per portion	net carbs per 100 g
Cream of chicken soup	1 mug	18	7
Cream of leek soup	1 mug	17	7
Cream of mushroom soup	1 mug	17	7
Cream of tomato soup	1 mug	20	9
Fish broth / bouillon	1 mug	0.5	1
Fish chowder	1 mug	11	4.5
Lobster bisque	1 mug	12	5
Minestrone soup	1 mug	15	6
Miso soup	1 mug	5.5	2.5
Potato chowder	1 mug	17	7
Potato Soup	1 mug	13	5
Tomato soup	1 mug	17	7
Vegetable broth / bouillon	1 mug	0.5	1
Vegetable soup	1 mug	23	9

SNACKS

Name	Portion size	Net carbs per Portion	Net carbs per 100 g
Almonds	20 nuts	2	5
Bagel	1 bagel	48	49
Biscuits	2 medium	14	68
Brazil nuts	10 nuts	3	4
Chocolate (dark)	44 g bar	24	55

Name	Portion size	Net carbs per Portion	Net carbs per 100 g
Chocolate (milk)	44 g bar	24	55
Chocolate (Tesco 85% dark)*	2 squares	0.5	3
Cookies	2 medium	14	68
Croissant	1 croissant	30	46
Doughnut	1 medium	22	50
Macadamia nuts	10 nuts	3	5
Mars bar	1 bar	30	60
Olives	10 large	2	2.8
Peanuts	1 large handful	3	8
Pecan nuts	10 halves	1.5	14
Peperami	1 stick	0.5	2.4
Pepperoni	any amount	0	0
Pitta bread	1 large	32	54
Popcorn	1 small container	60	61
Pork scratchings (rinds)	1 pack	0	0
Potato crisps (chips in US)	1 pack	14.5	50
Pretzels - hard	1 large	105	80
Pretzels - soft	1 large	96	70
Sandwich	1	26	31

* check net carbs on other 85% brands

DRINKS (alcoholic)

Pure spirits are okay, but all liqueurs are out, as are all sweetened drinks. You will stop burning fat while your body burns up the alcohol, so take it easy if you want to lose weight.

Drink	Drink size	Net carbs per drink
Amaretto	small measure	17
Baileys	small measure	5.5
Beer	1 can	13
Brandy	1 shot	0
Cognac	1 shot	0
Cointreau	small measure	10
Curacao	small measure	10
Drambuie	small measure	9
Galliano	small measure	8
Gin	1 shot	0
Grand Marnier	small measure	11
Kahlua	small measure	17
Red wine	1 glass	4
Rum	1 shot	0
Schnapps	small measure	12
Southern comfort	small measure	4
Tequila	1 shot	0
Triple sec	small measure	13
Vodka	1 shot	0
Whiskey	1 shot	0
White wine	1 glass	3

DRINKS (non-alcoholic)

Drink	Drink size	Net carbs per drink
Apple juice	200 ml glass	28
Cappuccino	1 mug	6
Coconut milk (unsweetened)	4 tablespoons	2
Coffee (black)	1 mug	0
Coffee (with dash of milk)	1 mug	0.5
Coke	1 can	35
Coke (diet)	1 can	0
Grapefruit juice	200 ml glass	18
Lemon juice	1 squeezed lemon	3.3
Lemonade	1 can	26
Lemonade (diet)	1 can	0
Milk (skimmed)	200 ml glass	12
Milk (whole)	200 ml glass	10
Milkshake	300 ml cup	60
Orange juice	200 ml glass	20
Pineapple juice	200 ml glass	30
Red Bull	250 ml can	27.5
Red Bull (sugar free)	250 ml can	0
Slush puppy ice	1 16oz glass	48
Tea (green)	1 mug	0
Tea with milk	1 mug	0.5
Tomato juice	200 ml glass	7.6
Water (carbonated)	200 ml glass	0
Water (still)	1 glass	0

DESSERTS

Name	Portion size	Net carbs per portion	Net carbs per 100 g
Apple pie	1 piece	38	33
Blueberries with cream	20 berries	4	14
Cheesecake	1 piece	20	25
Cherry pie	1 piece	43	38
Chocolate cake	1 piece	50	50
Cream (heavy /whipping)	2 tablespoons	1	2.7
Ice cream	1 individual	15	28
Raspberries*	10 large raspberries	3	6
Rice pudding	1 serving	25	21
Strawberries**	5 medium	3	6

* can vary in size, so weigh if in doubt
** great with cream

CONDIMENTS

Name	Portion size	Net Carbs per portion	Net carbs per 100 g
Almond nut butter	2 tablespoons	0	0
Capers	1 tablespoon	0.1	1.7
Chocolate spread	2 tablespoons	21	55
Cocoa powder	1 tablespoon	1	25
Garlic	1 clove	1	31
Gherkins	3 pickles	7	21
Herbs and spices	season to taste	0.1	1
Honey	1 tablespoon	17	82
Jam	1 tablespoon	13	68

Name	Portion size	Net Carbs per portion	Net carbs per 100 g
Maple syrup	1 tablespoon	13	68
Marmalade	1 tablespoon	13	66
Mayonnaise	2 tablespoons	0.2	0.6
Mayonnaise (light)*	2 tablespoons	3	9
Mustard	1 teaspoon	0.1	4
Olive oil	any amount	0	0
Olives	10 large	2	2.8
Peanut butter	2 tablespoons	4	14
Peanut butter (no added sugar)**	2 tablespoons	1	2.7
Pickled onions	4	1	5
Salt	teaspoon	0	0
Sesame oil	any amount	0	0
Splenda sweetener	1 teaspoon	0.5	97
Sugar	1 tablespoon	20	100
Tomato ketchup	2 tablespoons	5	26
Vinegar	any amount	0	0
Vinegar (balsamic)	2 tablespoons	5	17
Vinegar (cider)	2 tablespoons	0.2	0.9
Worcestershire sauce	1 tablespoon	3.3	19

*avoid low fat version

**check label (figures are for 'Whole Earth' brand)

Appendix B: Glycaemic Index of common foods

		Serving size (grams)	Glycaemic load per serving
Sponge cake, plain	46	63	17
Bagel, white	72	70	25
Baguette, white, plain	95	30	15
Hamburger bun	61	30	9
50% cracked wheat kernel bread	58	30	12
White wheat flour bread	71	30	10
Whole wheat bread, average in grain	71	30	9
Whole wheat bread, high in grain	51	30	7
Pitta bread, white	68	30	10
Corn tortilla	52	50	12
Wheat tortilla	30	50	8

DRINKS			
Coca Cola®, average	63	250 ml	16
Fanta®, orange soft drink	68	250 ml	23
Lucozade®, original	95±10	250 ml	40
Apple juice, unsweetened, average	44	250 ml	30
Orange juice, unsweetened	50	250 ml	12
Tomato juice, canned	38	250 ml	4
BREAKFAST CEREALS AND RELATED PRODUCTS			
All-Bran™, average	55	30	12
Coco Pops™, average	77	30	20
Cornflakes™, average	93	30	23
Muesli, average	66	30	16
Oatmeal, average	55	250	13
Instant oatmeal, average	83	250	30
Puffed wheat, average	80	30	17
Special K™	69	30	14
GRAINS			
Pearled barley, average	28	150	12
Sweet corn on the cob, average	60	150	20
Couscous, average	65	150	9
Quinoa	53	150	13
White rice	89	150	43

Quick cooking white basmati rice	67	150	28
Brown rice, average	50	150	16
Whole wheat kernels, average	30	50	11
Bulgur wheat, average	48	150	12
COOKIES AND CRACKERS			
Shortbread	64	25	10
Rice cakes, average	82	25	17
Rye crisps, average	64	25	11
Soda crackers	74	25	12
DAIRY PRODUCTS AND ALTERNATIVES			
Ice cream, regular	57	50	6
Ice cream, premium	38	50	3
Milk, full fat	41	250 ml	5
Milk, skimmed	32	250 ml	4
Reduced-fat yogurt with fruit, average	33	200	11
FRUITS			
Apple, average	39	120	6
Banana, ripe	62	120	16
Dates, dried	42	60	18
Grapefruit	25	120	3
Grapes, average	59	120	11
Orange, average	40	120	4
Peach, average	42	120	5
Peach, canned in light syrup	40	120	5
Pear, average	38	120	4
Prunes, pitted	29	60	10

130

Raisins	64	60	28
Watermelon	72	120	4
BEANS AND NUTS			
Baked beans, average	40	150	6
Blackeye peas, average	33	150	10
Black beans	30	150	7
Chickpeas, average	10	150	3
Chickpeas, canned in brine	38	150	9
Kidney beans, average	29	150	7
Lentils, average	29	150	5
Soy beans, average	15	150	1
Cashews, salted	27	50	3
Peanuts, average	7	50	0
PASTA and NOODLES			
Fettucini, average	32	180	15
Macaroni, average	47	180	23
Spaghetti, white, boiled, average	46	180	22
Spaghetti, wholemeal, boiled, average	42	180	17
SNACK FOODS			
Corn chips, plain, salted, average	42	50	11
M & M's®, peanut	33	30	6
Microwave popcorn, plain, average	55	20	6
Potato chips	51	50	12
Pretzels, oven-	83	30	16

131

baked			
Snickers® bar	51	60	18
VEGETABLES			
Green peas, average	51	80	4
Carrots, average	35	80	2
Parsnips	52	80	4
Baked russet potato, average	100	150	33
Boiled white potato, average	82	150	21
Instant mashed potato, average	87	150	17
Sweet potato, average	70	150	22
Yam, average	54	150	20
MISCELLANEOUS			
Hummus (chickpea salad dip)	6	30	0
Pizza, plain baked dough, served with parmesan cheese and tomato sauce	80	100	22
Honey, average	61	25	12

Appendix C: Recipe ideas

Here are a few low-carb recipe ideas. We hope they will give you some inspiration to experiment. You can see that there is no need to feel deprived. When you understand what foods you can eat, there are limitless delicious meal combinations you can come up with.

Chicken and Chorizo Salad

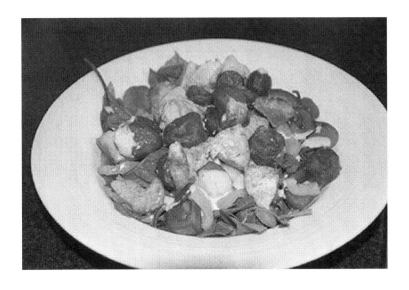

2 servings:

Diced chicken (as much as you like)
Chorizo, sliced (negligible carbs)
Salad leaves (lettuce, rocket, baby spinach)
2 tomatoes
8 slices cucumber
10 strips yellow pepper
1 avocado
Green olives
4 piquanté peppers stuffed with cream cheese (optional)
Caesar salad dressing

14 g net carbs per serving (10 g without the hot peppers)

Fry the chicken in a little olive oil in a pan. When nearly cooked, add the chorizo and cook for a few minutes until the oil runs out of the chorizo and coats the chicken. Place on top of the salad, season and add a little dressing.

Notes:

Waitrose and Sainsbury's own brands of Caesar salad dressing are fairly low in carbs, approx. 1–1.4 g net carbs per 15 ml serving. Check labels as some brands are much higher.

We used Peppadew peppers stuffed with cheese in oil for this dish. They come in a jar and, although they are quite expensive and not very low in carbs, two peppers each spices up a salad. Not something you should eat every day though. There are other brands (for example, Sainsbury's *Taste the Difference*) which are lower in carbs, and we will be buying these in the future.

You could also substitute the chicken with scallops (use a different dressing though) as they work very well with chorizo.

Tuna Niçoise Salad

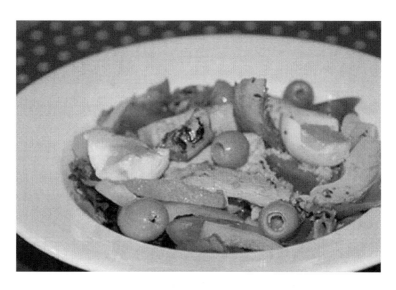

2 servings:

1 jar Albacore Tuna in extra virgin olive oil (or you can use tinned or fresh tuna)
2 tomatoes
8 thin slices cucumber
Mixed salad leaves
8 green pitted olives
2 hard-boiled eggs
1 small yellow pepper (or half a large one)
4 pieces chargrilled artichoke in olive oil
1 small avocado

Salad dressing (Newman's Own Family Recipe Italian Dressing is very low in carbs)

7.6 g net carbs per serving

Notes:
This is not a conventional niçoise salad, just a variation. You could replace the pepper with green beans and add anchovies if you wish.

Meatballs with Tomato Sauce and Vegetables

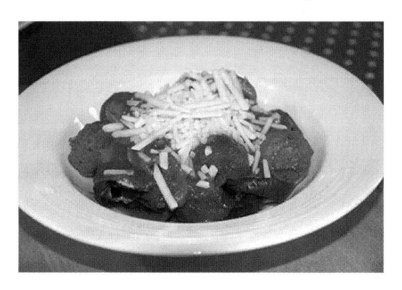

2 servings:

Ready-made meatballs or make your own with minced beef
2 medium-sized courgettes
1 medium aubergine
1 small shallot or 1 very small onion
2 cloves garlic
6 mushrooms (sliced)
200 g passata
100 g grated cheddar cheese
Thyme (1 teaspoon fresh or dried)
Salt and pepper

16 g net carbs per serving

Make the tomato sauce by frying the shallot/onion and garlic in a little olive oil, add the mushrooms and cook for a few minutes before adding the passata and thyme, and season with salt and pepper. Simmer on a low heat until cooked.

Place the meatballs on a baking tray. Slice the courgettes and aubergine, sprinkle with olive oil, season and put on a separate baking tray. Bake in a hot oven until the vegetables are slightly browned and the meatballs cooked through (approximately twenty minutes depending on your oven).

Layer the courgettes and aubergine in a pasta bowl (or plate), add the meatballs, then pour over the tomato sauce and sprinkle on the grated cheddar.

Notes:

Passata is relatively high in carbs, so do not use too much. Tinned chopped tomatoes are slightly lower, but again do not over use.

Portobello Mushroom with Poached Egg & Bacon

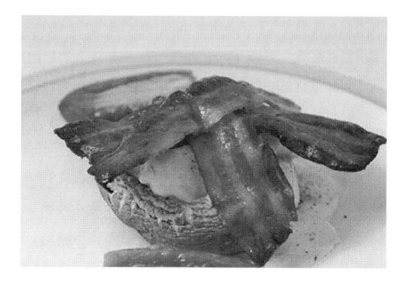

1 large Portobello mushroom or any large flat mushroom
1 egg (preferably free range)
4 rashers streaky bacon
1 tablespoon crème fraîche
A little olive oil
Salt and freshly ground black pepper

1. Pre-heat the oven to 200°C/400°F/Gas mark 6. Place the mushroom in a parcel of foil with a little olive oil and season with salt and pepper. Place on a baking tray and roast in the oven for about 20 minutes. You could grill the mushroom if you prefer.
2. Grill or cook the bacon in the oven until crisp.
3. Poach the egg.
4. Place the mushroom on a plate and add the egg on top with a spoonful of crème fraiche. Lay the bacon across or around the mushroom and egg and season with salt and pepper.

5 g net carbs

Notes:
This recipe is for one serving. Increase quantity for the number of people you wish to serve, or if you want more than one portion yourself!

Serve with a grilled plum tomato (approximately 1.7 net carbs) if you wish. You could also add some grated cheese on the mushroom as an extra ingredient. The carbs for this would be insignificant.

Ideal for breakfast, brunch or a light meal.

Beef Florentine

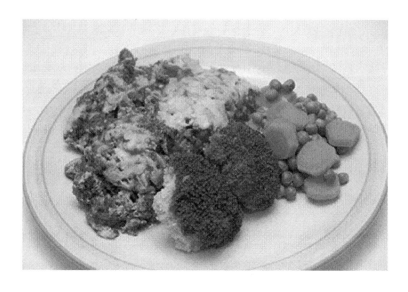

3 good-size servings:

500 g minced beef
1 tin chopped tomatoes
200 g pack button mushrooms
1 teaspoon dried oregano
2 cloves garlic (chopped or put through a garlic press)
150 g pack garlic and herb Boursin
200 g grated cheddar
260 g pack fresh spinach (or you could use frozen)
1 egg
2 heaped tablespoons milled flaxseed (optional, but gives a nice texture to the topping)
Salt and pepper

1.   Fry the mince for about 5 minutes, then add the garlic. Slice the mushrooms and add. Fry for a further 5 minutes, then add the chopped tomatoes

and oregano and season with salt and pepper. Cover and simmer on a low heat for about 30 minutes.

2. Cook the spinach and allow to cool. Squeeze as much water as you can from the spinach and roughly chop.

3. Beat the egg, then add 100 g of the grated cheddar, the Boursin and the spinach. Season and mix well.

4. Spread half of the beef mixture into an ovenproof dish. Top with the spinach and cheese mixture and then layer with the remaining beef.

5. Mix the flaxseed (if using) with the remaining 100g cheese and sprinkle on top of the mixture.

6. Cook in an oven preheated to 220°C/425°F/Gas mark 7 for about 25 minutes, until bubbling and golden brown.

8.7 g net carbs per serving

Notes:
Serve with broccoli, carrots and peas or vegetables of your choice from the recommended food list.

Lamb Steaks and Sausages with Vegetables

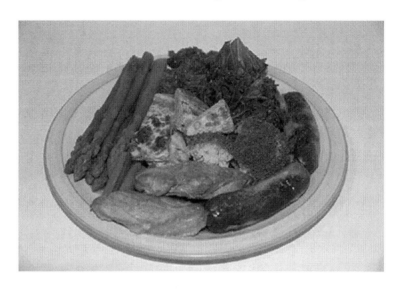

2 small lamb steaks per person
2 sausages per person (high meat content)
1 portion each of:
Asparagus
Sugar snap peas
Curly kale
Broccoli
Roasted swede:
Allow a quarter of swede per person. Cut into wedges, toss in olive oil, place on a baking sheet and sprinkle with dried thyme and season with salt and pepper. Bake in a hot oven 220°C/425°F/Gas mark 7 for about 40 minutes until soft and slightly browned. Gravy made with Bisto gravy granules for convenience. One 50 ml serving is 2.8 net carbs, so you can choose whether to add or not.

14 g net carbs per serving (without gravy)

Chicken Curry with
Cumin Spiced Cauliflower Rice

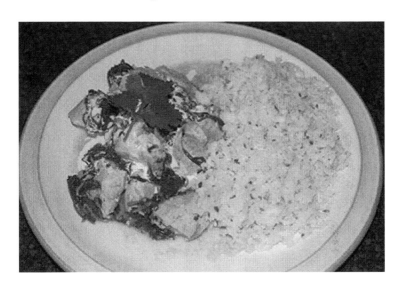

Serves 2:

400 g diced chicken
200 g fresh spinach
250 ml coconut cream
Fresh ginger (1 small piece, peeled)
2 cloves garlic
2 small red chillies
1 small shallot
2 tsp garam masala
½ tsp ground cumin
½ tsp ground turmeric
2 tbsp chopped fresh coriander
Salt and pepper
1 small cauliflower
1 tsp cumin seeds

11 g net carbs per serving

1. Crush the garlic and ginger to a paste and chop the shallot and chillies (deseed and remove the membrane if you want less heat).
2. Fry the chicken in a little olive oil until browned. Add the shallot, garlic, ginger and chillies and cook for a further couple of minutes. Stir in the garam masala, turmeric and ground cumin and cook for another minute.
3. Add the coconut cream, season and cook on a low heat for approximately 15–20 minutes.
4. In a separate saucepan, cook the spinach. Squeeze as much water out as you can. You can do this by allowing to cool enough to squeeze the water out by hand. Roughly chop.
5. Add the spinach and the chopped coriander to the chicken and stir in.
6. To make the cauliflower rice – cut out and discard the bottom core, then grate the cauliflower by hand or pulse in a food processor until it resembles rice. Place in a microwavable dish and stir in the cumin seeds. Season with a little salt, but do not add any water. Cook in a microwave oven on high for approximately 4 minutes (depending on the power of your microwave), stirring every minute. It should look fluffy and retain some texture, but not be 'mushy'.

Notes:

You can also add 1 tbsp of desiccated coconut to the curry when you add the coconut cream if you like.

Pork and Chorizo

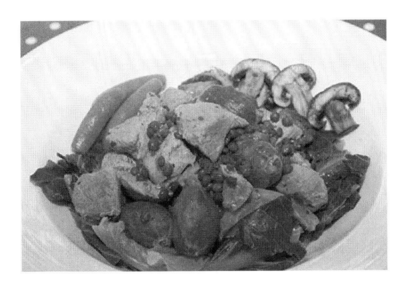

Serves 3-4

Cubed pork (about 200 g per person)
Pack mini chorizo cooking sausages or sliced chorizo
½ tsp dried sage
½ tsp dried thyme (or use fresh herbs if you have them)
1 large shallot or small onion cut into quarters
400 g tin puy lentils
400 g tin chicken consommé
1 Knorr chicken stockpot (optional, but adds extra flavour)
Spring greens
Mushrooms
Sugar snap peas

145

Approx. 12 g net carbs per serving (figure based on 3 servings)

Fry the pork in a little olive oil until browned. Add the sage and thyme and then the chicken consommé and stock pot. Bring to the boil and then turn the heat down and simmer until the stockpot has melted. Stir, then add the shallot or onion and season with some pepper and a little salt (chorizo is very salty so don't overdo it). Cover with a lid.

Place in the oven 160°C/320°F/Gas mark 3 for approximately one hour.

Add the chorizo and lentils and place back in the oven for a further thirty minutes or until the pork is tender.

Serve on a bed of boiled or steamed spring greens with some mushrooms and sugar snap peas.

Notes:

Instead of the chicken consommé, you can use 1 or 2 chicken stock cubes, or just the stockpot made up with water. You can also add 1 tbsp tomato puree. If you prefer a thicker gravy, you can use 1 tablespoon plain flour, but this will add 6g net carbs to the dish (2 g net carbs per person for three servings).

Sausages with Cauliflower Mash

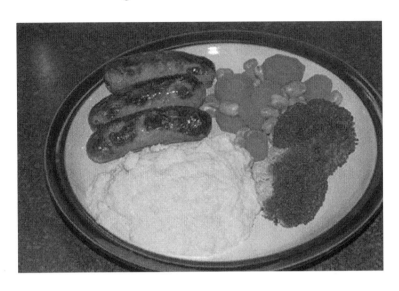

2 servings

6 good-quality pork sausages
1 small cauliflower
Knob of butter
2 tbsp double cream
2–3 tbsp grated cheddar cheese
4 florets broccoli
1 carrot
4 tbsp broad beans

14 g net carbs per serving

1. Grill or cook the sausages in the oven.
2. To make the cauliflower mash, boil the cauliflower until cooked. Season and add a knob of butter and the cream. Mash with a hand blender or use a food processor, adding the cheese when nearly done and mix in well. The cauliflower mash will be 'runnier'

than normal mash, but should still have a slightly firm consistency.

3.   Serve with broccoli, carrots and broad beans, or vegetables of your choice from the 'good food' list.

Notes:

If your daily intake of carbs allows, make a little bit of gravy to add to the sausages. You can also replace the cheddar cheese with parmesan if you prefer.

The sausages used for this dish were Paul Rankin, which are 85% pork. They work out to 1.2 g net carbs each sausage. If you have a large appetite you can add an extra sausage if you wish.

Cod Fillet with Ratatouille

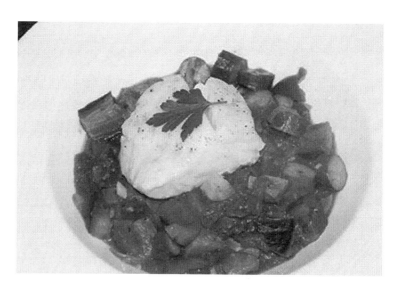

2 servings

2 cod fillets

2 courgettes

1 aubergine

½ fennel bulb

1 small green pepper

400 g tin chopped tomatoes

1 small onion or shallot

2 small fresh red chillies (optional)

2 cloves garlic

1 tsp dried oregano

Fresh basil (several leaves torn up)

1. Chop all the vegetables.
2. Heat some olive oil in a pan and fry the onion for a couple of minutes. Add the garlic and chillies (if using) and fry for another minute.
3. Add the courgettes, aubergine, fennel and green pepper and cook for a few minutes.
4. Pour in the chopped tomatoes. Stir and add the oregano and season with salt and pepper. Cover and simmer on a low heat for about 40 minutes (or cook on a low heat in the oven if preferred). Add the fresh basil at the end of the cooking time.
5. Drizzle a little olive oil over the cod and season with salt and pepper. Cook in the oven or pan fry. Be careful not to overcook.
6. Place the ratatouille in a dish and place the cod on top garnished with some fresh parsley.

15.5 g net carbs per serving

Notes:

Replace the fennel with two stalks of celery if you wish.

The chillies give a 'kick' to the ratatouille, but omit if you prefer it without.

Chocolate Brownies

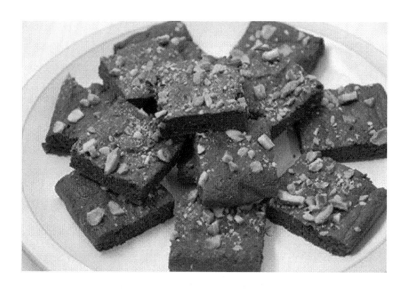

Makes 16 pieces

150 g (5½ oz) dark chocolate (85% cocoa solids)
100 g (3½ oz) butter
100 g (3½ oz) ground almonds
8 teaspoons granulated Splenda
4 eggs
1 tsp vanilla extract
25 g (1 oz) chopped pistachio nuts

1. Preheat the oven to 180°C/350°F/Gas mark 4. Line a 20 cm/8 inch square tin with baking parchment and grease.
2. In a heatproof bowl, melt the chocolate and butter by placing over a pan of simmering water. Stir occasionally until the chocolate and butter have melted.
3. Remove the bowl from the heat and stir in the vanilla extract. Leave to cool for a while and then add the ground almonds and Splenda and mix in well.
4. Separate the eggs. Lightly beat the egg yolks and stir into the chocolate mixture.
5. Whisk the egg whites until they form stiff peaks. Carefully fold one spoonful into the chocolate mixture and then fold in the rest until completely mixed in.
6. Spoon the mixture into the baking tin and sprinkle with the chopped pistachio nuts. Bake for 20-25 minutes until risen and firm on top, but still slightly gooey in the middle. Leave to cool in the tin, then turn out, remove baking parchment and cut into 16 pieces.

1.5 g (approx) net carbs per piece

Notes:
Enjoy as an occasional treat. It is **important that you use only 85%** dark chocolate for this recipe. The carbohydrate content is much lower than other dark chocolate and it has a high fibre content. Check package for carb content, as some brands vary.

You could also substitute the pistachio nuts with flaked almonds.

Walnut Loaf

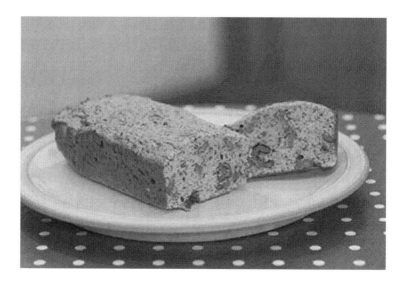

80g coconut flour (sifted)
40g milled flaxseed
1 tsp baking powder
4 eggs
2 tbsp Splenda
8 tbsp butter (melted)
150 ml milk
40 g walnuts (chopped)
Pinch of salt

1. Combine and mix all the dry ingredients together.
2. Add eggs, milk and butter and mix well.
3. Stir in the chopped walnuts.
4. Pour into a greased loaf pan or line with baking parchment.
5. Bake in the oven at 180°C/350°F/Gas mark 4 for approximately 40 minutes. Cover with foil if it looks like it's starting to burn on top.

36 g net carbs for the whole loaf – cuts into 6 slices, which equals 6g net carbs per slice

Notes:

We used lactose-free milk, which is lower in carbs than normal milk. We also used Tiana coconut flour which is quite expensive £5.99 for 500 g (you can buy it on Amazon and in health food shops), but a little goes a long way as the high-fibre content allows the flour to expand. The same with the flaxseed: we buy Linwoods Milled Organic Flaxseed, which again is expensive but lasts for ages.

Appendix D: Further Reading

Campbell S J 2012 *Low Carb Diet Strategies You Don't Know About* (Amazon Digital Services)

Campbell S J 2013 *Cardio Sucks! The Truth About Cardio & Weight Loss* (Amazon Digital Services)

Elliot R 2005 *The Vegetarian Low-Carb Diet* (Piatkus)

Ferriss T 2011 *The 4-Hour Body* (Ebury Digital)

Haakonson P, Haakonson H 2004 *Slow Carb For Life* (ECW Press)

Phinney S, Volek J 2011 *The Art And Science of Low Carbohydrate Living* (Beyond Obesity LLC)

Phinney S, Volek J 2012 *The Art And Science of Low Carbohydrate Performance* (Beyond Obesity LLC)

Taubes G 2010 *Why We Get Fat: And What to Do About It* (Anchor)

Waldron D 2014 *The Dissident Diet* (Amazon Digital Services)

Atkins R C 2003 *Dr Atkins New Diet Revolution* (Vermilion)

www.poundforpounddiet.co.uk

Printed in Great Britain
by Amazon

67908845R00097